THE
HEART DISEASE
PREVENTION
COOKBOOK

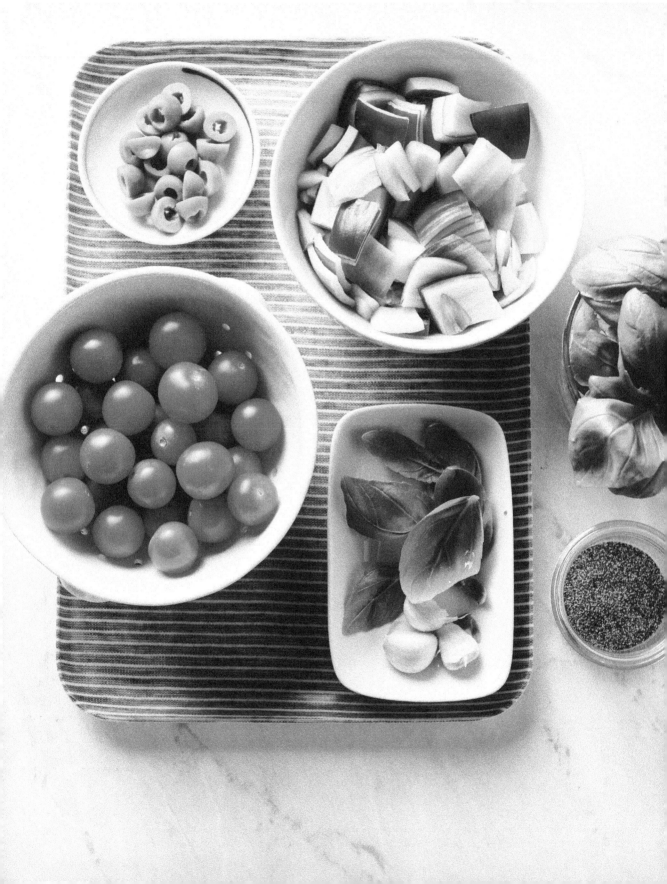

THE HEART DISEASE PREVENTION COOKBOOK

125 EASY MEDITERRANEAN DIET RECIPES FOR A HEALTHIER YOU

Cheryl Mussatto, MS, RD, LD

Photography by Marija Vidal

ROCKRIDGE
PRESS

To everyone
taking time to show their heart
some love.

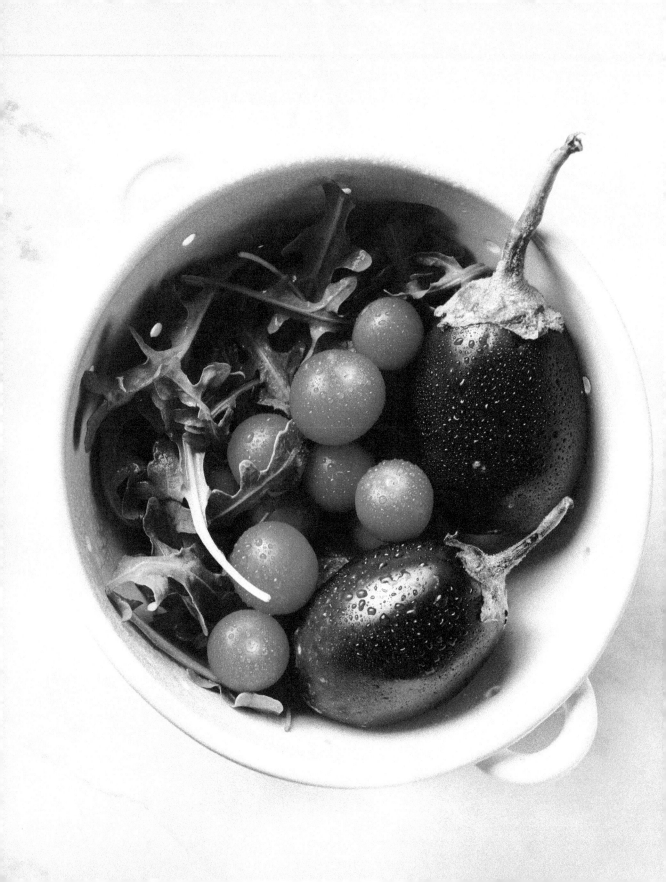

CONTENTS

INTRODUCTION

If you want to show your heart some love, start with your stomach! And you can begin your journey by following the dietary patterns of the Mediterranean region with this book, featuring recipes from countries such as Greece, Spain, Italy, and Morocco. Researchers and health professionals alike recommend the Mediterranean diet for heart health, as studies have shown that it helps reduce the risk of heart disease—not to mention it's pretty darn delicious.

Your heart is a fascinating organ. It continuously pumps oxygen- and nutrient-rich blood throughout your body to sustain life. This fist-sized powerhouse expands and contracts 100,000 times a day, pumping 5 to 6 quarts of blood each minute, or about 2,000 gallons per day.

As amazing as your heart is, your daily and long-term lifestyle habits have a huge impact on its health. Globally, heart disease is the number one cause of death. Heart disease is so common in the United States that few families have *not* had a loved one diagnosed with it. I remember the devastation of losing my beloved maternal grandmother, who died from a massive stroke, when I was 21. For years, she struggled with high blood pressure as her health suffered. While it was difficult to lose her, it also taught me that food choices matter. Ever since, my focus has remained on eating foods that promote heart health.

As a registered dietitian, I've worked with thousands of heart disease patients referred to me by doctors. Many of my clients believe a heart-healthy meal plan will be bland, boring, and difficult to follow. To their surprise, they discover how delicious and easy it is to plan, prepare, and enjoy Mediterranean-style meals. By ditching not-so-healthy dietary habits and embracing this way of eating, their blood pressure and lipid levels drop as their energy, vitality, and stamina soar.

Additionally, for nearly 20 years, I've been an adjunct professor at a community college, educating students on nutrition's role in reducing the risk of heart disease. No matter whom I'm coaching, I consider it a privilege to help others reach their health goals and live heart-healthy lives.

That's why I wholeheartedly endorse the Mediterranean diet. The multitude of studies supporting its ability to improve heart health and promote greater longevity is impressive. For years, it's been shown that people who blend the traditional flavors and cooking methods of the Mediterranean enjoy lower rates of heart disease.

So, let's begin your lifelong, heart-healthy journey of exploring an extraordinarily healthy and sustainable dietary pattern. Here's what this book offers:

• An explanation of heart disease and how diet and food can help prevent it

• Specific heart-healthy ingredients to have on demand, including red wine

• 125 easy, healthy, and creative recipes based on the Mediterranean diet that are affordable and use everyday ingredients

In short, this book is here to help you manage your heart health in the easiest and most delicious way possible. I want you to live life to its fullest without the burden of heart disease. I'll show you how while you discover why heart health matters.

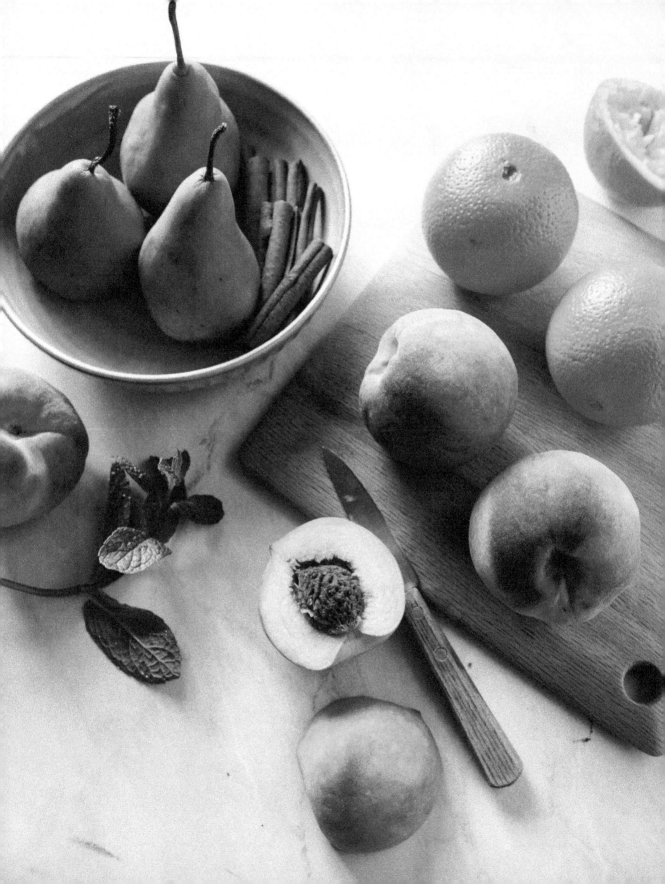

CHAPTER 1

PREVENT HEART DISEASE THROUGH FOOD

The heart is a symbol of love, but the sad reality is that most Americans don't give their heart the kind of love it deserves. Consider the fact that heart disease affects one in four Americans and is currently a leading cause of death. That's a sobering reality. However, by taking preventive steps such as following a heart-healthy diet, you can improve your chances of beating the odds.

Numerous studies have shown that the best plan for following a heart-healthy way of eating is the Mediterranean diet. While you may live thousands of miles from the Mediterranean, you can replicate the same healthy and nourishing dishes enjoyed in the region within your own home. This book introduces you to this style of eating with 125 easy and healthy recipes using the traditional flavors and cooking methods of the Mediterranean. Every day, my food choices reflect the principles of the Mediterranean diet: salad dressings made with extra-virgin olive oil and balsamic vinegar, fatty fish twice a week, beans and lentils added to soups, and fruit for dessert. As a registered dietitian working with patients on preventing heart disease, it's my hope you will also embrace this way of eating.

THE HEART TRUTH

In 1900, the leading cause of death in the United States was pneumonia, and the average life expectancy was 47 years. By 1930, the average life expectancy had risen to 60 years, and heart disease had become the number one cause of death. Ninety years later, heart disease is still the leading cause of death among Americans.

To understand heart disease, you need to know that it encompasses a wide range of conditions affecting your heart. The term *heart disease* is often used interchangeably with *cardiovascular disease*. Both terms refer to conditions that involve narrowed or blocked blood vessels, which can lead to a heart attack, severe chest pain (angina), or a stroke.

The beginnings of heart disease are evident when plaque, a waxy substance made up of cholesterol, fat, calcium, and other substances, develops in the arteries and blood vessels that lead to the heart. High blood pressure, elevated cholesterol or triglyceride levels, and cigarette smoking are common contributors to plaque accumulation. Plaque buildup narrows blood vessels, making your heart work harder to pump blood carrying necessary nutrients and oxygen throughout the body.

Like with all diseases, there are several risk factors involved in determining whether or not you are likely to develop heart disease. Two risk factors are out of your control: your age and your family history of heart disease. For women, the risk of heart disease increases around the age of 55, or at menopause, and for men, the risk begins earlier, at age 45. People from families with a high genetic risk for heart disease have almost double the likelihood of having a heart attack or stroke. The good news is they can lower their risk by almost half simply through leading a healthy lifestyle, such as having a heart-healthy diet.

Common risk factors for heart disease include the following:

• Obesity

• Insulin resistance or diabetes

• High total and LDL cholesterol levels and high triglycerides

• High blood pressure

• Physical inactivity

• Smoking

• An unhealthy diet

• High stress

• Sleep deprivation

• Excessive drinking

Most Common Types of Heart Disease

Here are the most common complications associated with heart disease:

• **Coronary artery disease:** This disease is caused by the blockage of one or more arteries that supply blood to the heart, usually due to atherosclerosis, which is a buildup of plaque that hardens and narrows artery walls.

• **Heart attack (myocardial infarction):** A heart attack occurs when there is an interruption in blood flow to the arteries supplying blood to the heart muscle caused by a blood clot that damages or destroys part of the heart muscle.

• **Stroke:** A form of cardiovascular disease, a stroke is the sudden death of brain cells due to lack of oxygen caused by the blockage of blood flow or the rupture of an artery to the brain.

• **Heart failure:** This is a condition in which the heart can't pump enough blood to meet the body's needs.

Beyond the Plate

Besides healthy food choices, lifestyle behaviors are also vital to lowering heart disease risk. Here are actionable steps you can take:

Quit smoking and avoid secondhand smoke. Smokers have twice the risk of developing heart disease and a higher death rate from heart attack. Nonsmokers exposed to secondhand smoke are also more likely to develop heart disease or lung cancer. Work with your doctor to quit smoking.

Monitor and manage blood pressure. Uncontrolled high blood pressure (130/80 mm Hg or higher) damages arteries, leading to plaque buildup that increases the likelihood of blood clots. Have your blood pressure checked at least yearly, and follow your doctor's treatment plan to reduce it if necessary.

Be physically active. Regular exercise leads to a healthier body weight, reduces high blood pressure, and stimulates good blood circulation. At least 150 minutes per week of moderate-intensity aerobic activity or 75 minutes per week of vigorous aerobic activity is recommended by the American Heart Association.

Reach and maintain a healthy body weight. A healthy body weight allows better blood circulation with less strain on your heart.

Control diabetes. Diabetes increases the risk of heart disease. Get tested and work with your doctor to manage diabetes with diet, exercise, and medication.

Manage stress. Long-term stress can increase your heart rate and blood pressure, damaging artery walls. Reduce stress and increase endorphin release through meditation, yoga, and exercise.

Limit alcohol. Too much alcohol can raise blood pressure, cause cardiomyopathy, and increase your risk of stroke while also increasing triglyceride levels and causing irregular heartbeats.

THE MEDITERRANEAN DIET AND HEART HEALTH

Life is about choices. These choices include what to wear, when to go to bed at night, and what to eat. It's our food choices that have a direct impact on heart health. When you make every bite count with healthy choices, your heart will reap the benefits.

Since the 1960s, studies have found that people living in countries bordering the Mediterranean Sea—such as Greece, Italy, Morocco, Sicily, and Spain—had longer life spans and lower rates of coronary heart disease. Scientific research has routinely shown that the Mediterranean style of eating is consistent with keeping the heart healthy. That's why both the Dietary Guidelines for Americans and the World Health Organization recognize the Mediterranean diet as a healthy and sustainable way of eating that promotes physical well-being while reducing heart disease.

The PREDIMED study, a well-known randomized clinical trial whose results were published in 2013 and reanalyzed in 2018, supports Mediterranean dietary patterns. Researchers followed over 7,000 women and men in Spain for almost five years to study the impact the Mediterranean diet had on cardiovascular disease. Results showed that the Mediterranean diet reduced risk for heart events by 30 percent when compared to a low-fat diet. Thanks to years of continued research on the impact of the Mediterranean diet on heart health, people everywhere can take steps to reduce their risk of developing heart disease.

Benefits of the Mediterranean Diet

While there is no single definition of the Mediterranean diet, it is typically high in vegetables, fruits, whole grains, beans, nuts, seeds, and olive oil, along with fatty fish. This liberal use of plant-based foods means a diet rich in fiber, antioxidants, phytochemicals, and vitamins and minerals—everything you need for improving heart health.

The benefits of following a Mediterranean diet should be crystal clear. Filling your plate with predominantly plant-based foods and moderate servings of fish, poultry, and dairy helps reduce plaque formation, blood pressure, inflammation, and formation of clots. With less plaque buildup and reduced blood pressure, your heart has an easier workload.

Foods abundant in a wide variety of nutrients are smart for heart health. Not only is eating Mediterranean-style meals appetizing to your taste buds, but you'll also be consuming heart-friendly foods rich in nutrients such as potassium, magnesium, folate, calcium, and omega-3 fatty acids.

While primarily known for benefiting heart health, following the Mediterranean diet may also do the following:

- Prevent cognitive decline leading to dementia

- Help with weight loss and maintenance

- Help manage type 2 diabetes

- Relieve symptoms of rheumatoid arthritis

Heart-Healthy Nutrients

Potassium and magnesium: These minerals are found predominately in dark leafy greens, whole grains, and nuts—all Mediterranean diet staples—and help regulate blood pressure, a major risk factor for heart disease.

Folate: This B vitamin regulates homocysteine in the blood. High levels of homocysteine may damage blood vessel walls and promote blood clots. The Mediterranean diet emphasizes rich sources of folate, such as whole-grain breads and cereals, avocados, and oranges.

Calcium: Well-known for building bone, calcium benefits heart health, too. By regulating weight management and blood pressure, calcium indirectly keeps your ticker running smoothly. Good sources of calcium include dairy foods, almonds, and broccoli, all part of the Mediterranean diet.

Monounsaturated fats: These heart-healthy fats come from fish oils; extra-virgin olive oil; certain nuts, like hazelnuts, almonds, and pecans; and seed oils, such as canola, peanut, and flaxseed. Their heart-healthy secret is attributed to bioactive polyphenols, powerful anti-inflammatory substances that help protect heart health.

Omega-3 fatty acids: A heart-healthy diet is not complete without omega-3 fatty acids, abundant in fatty fish, a staple of the Mediterranean diet. Valuable sources of omega-3s include salmon, albacore tuna, trout, mackerel, sardines, and anchovies, along with flaxseed and walnuts. Omega-3s have numerous benefits, such as lowering triglyceride levels and blood pressure, reducing the growth rate of artery-clogging plaque, and preventing the formation of clots and inflammation within the blood vessels.

Basics for Your Heart

Listed next are foods to enjoy and foods to avoid for optimal heart health.

Foods to Enjoy

- **Leafy greens/vegetables and fiber-rich fruits:** These powerhouses make up a majority of the diet, with the recommended consumption of four or more servings a day of vegetables and three or more servings of fruit.

- **Whole grains:** Whole-grain bread, cereal, and pasta and other whole grains, such as farro and bulgur, are excellent sources of fiber, which helps improve blood cholesterol levels while reducing risk of heart disease. Enjoy four or more servings daily.

- **Legumes, nuts, and seeds:** Rich in minerals and fiber without unhealthy saturated fats, legumes such as lentils, peas, and beans, along with nuts and seeds, should be consumed three or more times a week.

- **Fish rich in omega-3 fatty acids:** Twice a week, plan a meal of omega-3-rich fish, such as fresh or water-packed tuna, salmon, trout, herring, mackerel, anchovies, or sardines, to reduce your risk of heart disease and stroke.

- **Healthy fats:** Have 4 tablespoons or more each day by using extra-virgin olive oil in cooking and salad dressings, or choose avocado or natural peanut butter instead of butter or margarine.

- **Low-fat dairy:** Daily or weekly, enjoy low to moderate amounts of nonfat or low-fat Greek or plain yogurt and skim or 1 percent milk. Small amounts of natural cheeses, such as Brie, feta, or ricotta, are okay, too.

- **Eggs and poultry:** There is no limit on fat-free egg whites, but eat egg yolks in moderation. Choose skinless white-meat poultry that is baked, broiled, or grilled once or twice a week.

- **Lean red meat:** Limit your intake to a 3-ounce portion of loin or round cuts of meat (e.g., tenderloin or top round steak) no more than once a week.

- **Herbs and spices:** Use these meal-enhancing flavor boosters daily to reduce your use of salt and sugar.

Foods to Avoid

- **Pastries, sodas, and candies:** These sugary treats have little nutritional value.

- **Refined grains:** Bread, pasta, and pizza dough made with white flour lack the fiber necessary to lower blood cholesterol or help you maintain a healthy weight.

- **Saturated fats:** Unhealthy saturated fats can increase the risk of heart disease. These fats include butter, sour cream, animal fat, full-fat dairy, and tropical oils like coconut and palm oils.

- **Processed meats:** Cold cuts, sausage, hot dogs, and bacon are associated with an elevated risk of heart disease.

- **Fried foods:** Foods such as chicken, fish, or chips that have been fried not only add extra calories, increasing weight gain, but may also increase the risk of dying from a heart-related issue.

Red Wine Explainer

Most followers of the Mediterranean diet enjoy a glass or two of red wine daily, but that's it. Slowly sipping a glass of heart-healthy wine with a meal—never on an empty stomach—is the right approach. Consuming red wine with food helps slow the absorption of alcohol, aids in digestion, and minimizes inflammation in blood vessels.

A polyphenol called resveratrol is red wine's secret ingredient. Resveratrol is believed to promote heart health by protecting blood vessel linings, lowering levels of LDL or "bad" cholesterol, reducing inflammation, and preventing blood clots.

Moderation is key when consuming any beverage containing alcohol. Women can have one glass (5 ounces) of red wine a day, while men are allowed up to two glasses a day. The Mediterranean diet does not require drinking wine or any alcohol. In fact, drinking grape juice made from Concord grapes and eating purple grapes provide similar benefits.

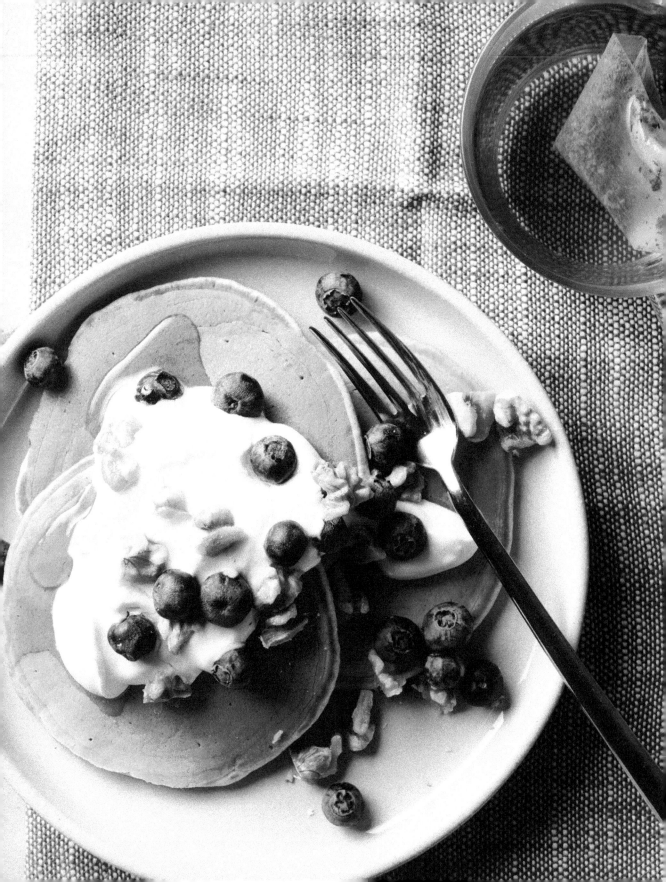

CHAPTER 2

BREAKFASTS AND BEVERAGES

< *Greek Yogurt Pancakes with
Yogurt and Honey Topping,
page 16*

CHIA BERRY SMOOTHIE

GLUTEN-FREE, VEGETARIAN

Serves 2 | Prep time: 15 minutes | Serving size: 2 cups

Fast, easy, filling, nutritious, and delicious. If that sounds like something you'd like to have for breakfast, then this smoothie will be a real treat. Loaded with vitamin C–rich berries, this thick and delicious breakfast smoothie makes the perfect on-the-go weekday meal.

2 cups skim milk

2 tablespoons chia seeds

2 cups frozen mixed berries (sugar-free)

¼ cup nonfat plain Greek yogurt

1 tablespoon honey (optional)

In a blender, combine the milk, chia seeds, berries, yogurt, and honey (if using), and blend until smooth. Serve.

Substitution tip: Make this vegan by replacing the milk with your favorite plain nondairy milk and using a vegan yogurt, such as plain cashew yogurt. Don't forget to omit the honey in your vegan variation!

Per Serving: Calories: 229; Total fat: 3g; Saturated fat: <1g; Cholesterol: 5mg; Carbohydrates: 35g; Fiber: 8g; Protein: 15g; Sodium: 129mg

ORANGE-SPINACH SMOOTHIE

ALLERGEN-FREE, GLUTEN-FREE, VEGETARIAN

Serves 2 | Prep time: 5 minutes | Serving size: 1½ cups

Get your heart-healthy greens at breakfast by adding a little bit of spinach to a juicy orange–flavored smoothie. Fresh-squeezed juice works best here, but you can also enjoy this smoothie with store-bought orange juice, although the flavors won't be as vibrant.

1 cup skim milk

1½ cups fresh-squeezed orange juice

1 teaspoon peeled grated fresh ginger or ground turmeric

3 cups baby spinach

1 tablespoon honey (optional)

In a blender, combine the milk, orange juice, ginger, spinach, and honey (if using), and blend until smooth. Serve.

Nutritional boost: Boost omega-3 fatty acids by adding ¼ cup of chopped walnuts to the smoothie before you blend it.

Per Serving: Calories: 141; Total fat: 1g; Saturated fat: <1g; Cholesterol: 3mg; Carbohydrates: 28g; Fiber: 2g; Protein: 7g; Sodium: 106mg

BLUEBERRY, YOGURT, AND PEPITA BREAKFAST PARFAITS

ALLERGEN-FREE, GLUTEN-FREE, VEGETARIAN

Serves 2 | Prep time: 5 minutes | Serving size: 2½ cups

These nutritional-powerhouse yogurt parfaits have a hint of sweetness, creamy Greek yogurt, juicy antioxidant-rich berries, and pepitas (hulled pumpkin seeds) for crunch. Layer them as pretty as you please, but if you'd rather just dump everything in a bowl, nobody will judge you!

2 cups nonfat plain Greek yogurt

1 teaspoon grated orange zest, plus more for garnish

2 tablespoons honey

½ teaspoon ground cinnamon

1 cup fresh blueberries, divided

4 tablespoons pepitas, divided

1. In a small bowl, whisk together the yogurt, orange zest, honey, and cinnamon.
2. In each of two parfait glasses, spoon in ½ cup of the yogurt mixture.
3. Add ¼ cup of blueberries to each and sprinkle with 1 tablespoon of pepitas.
4. Spoon another ¼ cup of the yogurt mixture into each parfait.
5. Layer with another ¼ cup of blueberries each. Top with the remaining yogurt.
6. Sprinkle each with the remaining 1 tablespoon of pepitas and add a bit of finely grated orange zest for garnish before serving.

Ingredient tip: Use a rasp-style grater to get the perfect orange zest. When zesting, make sure you get only the orange part and not the white part (pith), which can impart bitter flavors.

Per Serving: Calories: 327; Total fat: 8g; Saturated fat: 1g; Cholesterol: 0mg; Carbohydrates: 38g; Fiber: 3g; Protein: 28g; Sodium: 148mg

EASY APPLE-CINNAMON OATS

VEGETARIAN

Serves 4 | Prep time: 5 minutes | Cook time: 25 minutes | Serving size: ½ cup

Oats are a great way to start your day because they stick to your ribs and provide a sustained boost of fiber-rich complex carbohydrates. This recipe is the grown-up version of those instant oatmeal packets you probably ate as a kid—only they taste better and they're better for you.

1½ cups water

1½ cups unsweetened apple juice

½ cup skim milk

Pinch salt

1 cup steel-cut oats

½ cup chopped dried apples

1 teaspoon ground cinnamon

1 cup nonfat plain Greek yogurt

2 tablespoons pure maple syrup

1. In a medium pot, bring the water, apple juice, milk, and salt to a boil over medium-high heat.

2. Stir in the oats, dried apples, and cinnamon. Bring to a boil, stirring.

3. Reduce the heat to low. Simmer, stirring occasionally, for about 20 minutes, or until the oats are soft.

4. In a small bowl, whisk together the yogurt and syrup. Stir into the oatmeal and serve.

Substitution tip: You can make this vegan by using an unflavored, unsweetened nondairy milk and omitting the Greek yogurt. Instead, drizzle the maple syrup right over the top of the oatmeal with a little extra nondairy milk if desired.

Per Serving: Calories: 278; Total fat: 3g; Saturated fat: 1g; Cholesterol: 1mg; Carbohydrates: 56g; Fiber: 5g; Protein: 13g; Sodium: 78mg

GREEK YOGURT PANCAKES WITH YOGURT AND HONEY TOPPING

VEGETARIAN

Serves 4 | Prep time: 10 minutes | Cook time: 15 minutes | Serving size: 3 pancakes

Who doesn't love pancakes? These have a little extra protein, so they'll stick with you longer. The secret ingredient is calcium-rich Greek yogurt, which adds a boost of protein while keeping the pancakes moist and light.

1 cup whole-wheat flour

1 cup white flour

¼ teaspoon sea salt

3 teaspoons baking powder

½ teaspoon ground cinnamon

1 cup skim milk

4 tablespoons honey, divided

Zest and juice of 1 orange

2 eggs, lightly beaten

1 teaspoon pure vanilla extract

1½ cups nonfat plain Greek yogurt, divided

Nonstick cooking spray

1. In a medium bowl, whisk together the whole-wheat flour, white flour, salt, baking powder, and cinnamon.

2. In another bowl, whisk together the milk, 2 tablespoons of honey, orange zest and juice, eggs, vanilla, and ½ cup of yogurt.

3. Add the wet ingredients to the dry ingredients and fold until just combined.

4. Spray a skillet with nonstick cooking spray and heat over medium-high heat.

5. Working in batches, ladle ¼ cup of batter for each pancake into the pan. Cook on one side until bubbles form, about 3 minutes. Flip and cook until the other side is done, about 2 minutes more.

6. While the pancakes cook, in a small bowl, whisk together the remaining 2 tablespoons of honey and the remaining 1 cup of yogurt.

7. Serve the pancakes with the yogurt spooned on top.

Nutrition boost: You can top these with up to ¼ cup of chopped walnuts for added crunch and a boost of omega-3 fatty acids.

Per Serving: Calories: 381; Total fat: 3g; Saturated fat: 1g; Cholesterol: 94mg; Carbohydrates: 70g; Fiber: 5g; Protein: 21g; Sodium: 472mg

MAPLE FARRO HOT CEREAL WITH DRIED APRICOTS

ALLERGEN-FREE, VEGAN

Serves 4 | **Prep time: 5 minutes** | **Cook time: 25 minutes** | **Serving size: ½ cup**

No Mediterranean diet is complete without a delicious, hearty grain such as farro. A great alternative to oatmeal, farro takes only a few minutes to cook. Dried apricots and a hint of maple syrup add just the right amount of sweetness to get your day started right.

1 cup water

1½ cups unsweetened apple juice

1 cup farro

Pinch sea salt

3 tablespoons pure maple syrup

½ cup chopped dried apricots

¼ cup chopped walnuts or pecans (optional)

1. In a small pot, combine the water, apple juice, farro, and sea salt.
2. Heat the pot over medium-high heat and bring the mixture to a boil, stirring occasionally, then reduce the heat to medium-low.
3. Simmer, stirring occasionally, until the farro is tender, about 20 minutes.
4. Remove from the heat. Stir in the syrup, apricots, and nuts (if using), and serve.

Ingredient tip: You can also make this overnight in the slow cooker so it's ready to go in the morning. Just combine the water, juice, farro, and salt in a slow cooker, cover, and cook on low for 8 hours. Stir in the syrup, apricots, and nuts in the morning.

Per Serving: Calories: 290; Total fat: 1g; Saturated fat: 0g; Cholesterol: 0mg; Carbohydrates: 66g; Fiber: 6g; Protein: 8g; Sodium: 36mg

MEDITERRANEAN-STYLE VEGGIE AND EGG SCRAMBLE

GLUTEN-FREE, VEGETARIAN

Serves 4 | Prep time: 10 minutes | Cook time: 10 minutes | Serving size: ½ cup

It doesn't take long to scramble eggs for your morning breakfast, so this works even for weekdays. The veggies add tons of flavor and texture, so this uniquely delicious scrambled egg breakfast is destined to become a family favorite.

2 tablespoons extra-virgin olive oil

½ red onion, chopped

½ red bell pepper, seeded and chopped

½ small zucchini, chopped

1 cup cherry tomatoes, halved

8 eggs, beaten

½ teaspoon dried oregano

½ teaspoon sea salt

¼ teaspoon freshly ground black pepper

1 garlic clove, minced

1. In a large nonstick skillet, heat the olive oil over medium-high heat until it shimmers.
2. Add the onion, bell pepper, zucchini, and tomatoes. Cook, stirring occasionally, until the vegetables begin to brown, about 5 minutes.
3. While the vegetables cook, in a medium bowl, whisk together the eggs, oregano, salt, and black pepper, and set aside.
4. Add the garlic to the vegetables in the skillet and cook, stirring constantly, for 30 seconds.
5. Add the egg mixture and cook, stirring, until the eggs are set, about 4 minutes more. Serve hot.

Variation tip: You can add ¼ cup of crumbled feta cheese as garnish. Sprinkle it on after the eggs are cooked.

Per Serving: Calories: 225; Total fat: 17g; Saturated fat: 4g; Cholesterol: 372mg; Carbohydrates: 6g; Fiber: 1g; Protein: 14g; Sodium: 438mg

MEDITERRANEAN-SPICED SWEET POTATO HASH WITH FRIED EGG

GLUTEN-FREE, VEGETARIAN

Serves 4 | Prep time: 10 minutes | Cook time: 15 minutes | Serving size: ½ cup hash and 1 egg

Warm spices take a simple breakfast hash from basic to beautiful, so this dish will definitely liven up your morning. Topping it with a fried egg makes it not only nice to look at but even nicer to eat.

3 tablespoons extra-virgin olive oil, divided

½ red onion, chopped

½ red bell pepper, seeded and chopped

2 sweet potatoes, peeled and cut into ½-inch cubes

½ teaspoon ground coriander

½ teaspoon dried oregano

½ teaspoon ground allspice

½ teaspoon sea salt, plus more for seasoning

4 eggs

Freshly ground black pepper

1. In a large nonstick skillet, heat 2 tablespoons of olive oil over medium-high heat until it shimmers.

2. Add the onion, bell pepper, potatoes, coriander, oregano, allspice, and ½ teaspoon of salt. Cook, stirring occasionally, until the potatoes are browned and soft, about 10 minutes.

3. While the vegetables are cooking, in another large nonstick pan, heat the remaining 1 tablespoon of olive oil over low heat for 2 minutes.

4. Carefully crack the eggs into the pan, and season them with just a sprinkle of salt and black pepper. Cook, undisturbed, until the eggs are set, about 3 minutes.

5. Turn off the heat. Carefully flip the eggs. Allow the eggs to rest in the pan for 30 seconds.

6. Serve the eggs on top of the hash.

Nutritional boost: Add some nutritious leafy greens to this dish. After the potatoes are browned, add 2 cups of baby spinach and cook, stirring, until soft and wilted, about 2 minutes.

Per Serving: Calories: 241; Total fat: 16g; Saturated fat: 3g; Cholesterol: 186mg; Carbohydrates: 19g; Fiber: 3g; Protein: 8g; Sodium: 371mg

SALMON AND TOMATO FRITTATA

GLUTEN-FREE

Serves 4 | Prep time: 10 minutes | Cook time: 10 minutes | Serving size: ¼ of the frittata

This frittata is delicious any time of the year, but it's really elevated in the summer, when fresh tomatoes are in season. You can use any type of cooked salmon. It's a great way to use leftover fish. If using canned salmon, drain and rinse it to remove any excess salt from processing.

2 tablespoons extra-virgin olive oil

½ onion, finely chopped

1 cup cherry tomatoes, halved

2 garlic cloves, minced

1 cup flaked cooked salmon

Zest of 1 lemon

6 eggs, beaten

1 teaspoon dried dill

½ teaspoon sea salt

¼ teaspoon freshly ground black pepper

¼ cup crumbled feta cheese

1. Preheat the oven's broiler on high.
2. In a large ovenproof skillet, heat the olive oil over medium-high heat until it shimmers.
3. Add the onion and tomatoes and cook, stirring occasionally, until the onion is soft, about 4 minutes.
4. Add the garlic and cook, stirring constantly, for 30 seconds.
5. Add the salmon and lemon zest and cook for 1 minute.
6. In a large bowl, whisk together the eggs, dill, salt, and pepper.
7. Remove the skillet from the heat and spread the veggies and salmon in an even layer on the bottom of the skillet. Carefully pour the eggs over the vegetables and salmon and sprinkle with the feta cheese.
8. Broil until the top puffs and the cheese melts, 2 to 3 minutes. Let cool slightly before serving.

Substitution tip: If you're allergic to dairy, you can still enjoy this frittata—simply omit the feta cheese.

Per Serving: Calories: 265; Total fat: 19g; Saturated fat: 5g; Cholesterol: 309mg; Carbohydrates: 5g; Fiber: 1g; Protein: 19g; Sodium: 524mg

SPINACH, ROASTED RED PEPPER, HUMMUS, AND FETA OMELET

GLUTEN-FREE, VEGETARIAN

Serves 4 | **Prep time: 10 minutes** | **Cook time: 15 minutes** | **Serving size: ¼ of the omelet**

The great thing about omelets is that you can wrap them around any vegetable or meat filling and you've got a hearty breakfast. This omelet has classically delicious Mediterranean flavors and a colorful filling.

3 tablespoons extra-virgin olive oil, divided

3 cups baby spinach

1 garlic clove, minced

½ (16-ounce) jar roasted red peppers, drained and patted dry

1 tablespoon capers, drained and rinsed

6 eggs, beaten

½ teaspoon sea salt

¼ teaspoon freshly ground black pepper

¼ cup Easy Hummus (page 32) or store-bought hummus

¼ cup crumbled feta cheese

1. In a large nonstick skillet, heat 2 tablespoons of olive oil over medium-high heat until it shimmers.

2. Add the baby spinach and cook, stirring occasionally, until it is wilted and soft, about 3 minutes.

3. Add the garlic and cook, stirring constantly, for 30 seconds.

4. Add the roasted red peppers and capers and cook, stirring until just heated, about 1 minute more.

5. While the vegetables cook, in a medium bowl, whisk together the eggs, salt, and black pepper.

6. Remove the vegetables from the skillet and set them aside. Wipe out the skillet with a paper towel and return it to the heat over medium-high heat.

7. Pour in the remaining 1 tablespoon of olive oil and heat it until it shimmers, swirling the skillet to coat the bottom.

8. Add the eggs and allow them to cook without stirring, until the edges are firm, 2 to 3 minutes.

9. Using a silicone spatula, carefully pull the set eggs away from the edges of the pan. Tilt the pan to allow uncooked eggs to flow into the spaces you made.

continued >

10. Continue cooking without stirring until the omelet is set, another 3 to 4 minutes.

11. Reduce the heat to low. Carefully spread the hummus on half of the omelet. Spoon the vegetables over the hummus and sprinkle with the feta cheese.

12. Fold the omelet in half. Cover and cook for about 1 minute to allow the cheese to melt. Serve.

Variation tip: Not big on folding omelets? Keep your cooked veggies in the skillet and add the eggs. Cook, scrambling, for about 3 minutes. Sprinkle with the feta cheese, turn off the heat, cover, and allow the cheese to melt for 1 minute. Spoon the hummus over the top before serving.

Per Serving: Calories: 278; Total fat: 23g; Saturated fat: 6g; Cholesterol: 287mg; Carbohydrates: 7g; Fiber: 2g; Protein: 13g; Sodium: 653mg

CAPRESE BREAKFAST WRAPS

VEGETARIAN

Serves 2 | Prep time: 10 minutes | Cook time: 5 minutes | Serving size: 1 wrap

This breakfast wrap is packed with vibrant, fresh flavors from basil and tomatoes. It's good all year round but especially in the summer. If you have access to fresh, homegrown tomatoes and basil, grab them and use them for this wrap. You'll be glad you did.

2 tablespoons extra-virgin olive oil

4 eggs, beaten

¼ teaspoon sea salt

Pinch freshly ground black pepper

2 large soft whole-wheat tortillas

1 cup cherry tomatoes, quartered

4 mini balls fresh mozzarella, quartered

¼ cup chopped fresh basil

1. In a large nonstick skillet, heat the olive oil over medium-high heat until it shimmers.
2. Add the eggs, salt, and pepper and stir until scrambled, about 5 minutes.
3. Wrap the tortillas in a damp paper towel and warm them in the microwave on high for about 30 seconds.
4. Divide the eggs between the tortillas and top with the tomatoes, mozzarella, and basil. Roll into wraps and serve immediately.

Per Serving: Calories: 531; Total fat: 33g; Saturated fat: 9g; Cholesterol: 383mg; Carbohydrates: 39g; Fiber: 2g; Protein: 21g; Sodium: 860mg

ON-THE-GO MEZZE BREAKFAST PITA

GLUTEN-FREE, VEGETARIAN

Serves 2 | Prep time: 10 minutes | Serving size: 2 pita halves

If you adore mezze platters, you can have them for breakfast, too. This breakfast pita goes with you, it's fast and easy to prepare, and it's like carrying your mezze platter in a handy pocket. What could be better?

2 tablespoons extra-virgin olive oil

1 tablespoon red wine vinegar

1 garlic clove, minced

½ teaspoon Dijon mustard

¼ teaspoon sea salt

⅛ teaspoon freshly ground black pepper

3 hard-boiled eggs, chopped (see Ingredient tip)

½ (12-ounce) jar roasted red peppers, drained and patted dry

½ cup cherry tomatoes, halved

3 cups baby spinach

2 whole-wheat pitas, halved

½ cup White Bean Dip (page 66)

1. In a small bowl, whisk together the olive oil, red wine vinegar, garlic, mustard, salt, and black pepper to make a vinaigrette.
2. In a large bowl, combine the eggs, roasted red peppers, tomatoes, and baby spinach.
3. Toss with the vinaigrette.
4. Spread the inside of each pita half with 2 tablespoons of white bean dip.
5. Divide the salad between the pita halves and serve.

Ingredient tip: To hard-boil eggs, place the eggs in a single layer in the bottom of a pot. Cover them with water so the water is 1 inch over the top of the eggs. Put the pot over high heat and bring to a boil. As soon as the water boils, turn off the heat and cover the pot. Allow the eggs to sit in the hot water for 14 minutes. Plunge the eggs into an ice bath (ice and cold water) to stop cooking.

Per Serving: Calories: 520; Total fat: 27g; Saturated fat: 5g; Cholesterol: 279mg; Carbohydrates: 51g; Fiber: 7g; Protein: 20g; Sodium: 839mg

ENGLISH MUFFIN BREAKFAST PIZZA

Serves 4 | **Prep time: 10 minutes** | **Cook time: 15 minutes** | **Serving size: 1 pizza**

Pizza for breakfast? Why not? English muffins make the perfect pizza crust. Because your crust is already baked, these tasty treats cook quickly and easily, and they're popular with the kiddos as well.

1 tablespoon extra-virgin olive oil

4 ounces turkey ham, finely chopped

4 eggs, beaten

¼ teaspoon sea salt

½ cup canned crushed tomatoes with basil, drained

½ (12-ounce) jar roasted red peppers, drained

1 garlic clove, minced

4 English muffins, split and toasted

½ cup shredded mozzarella cheese

1. Preheat the oven to 400°F. Line a baking sheet with parchment paper.
2. In a medium nonstick skillet, heat the olive oil over medium-high heat until it shimmers.
3. Add the turkey ham and cook, stirring, for 2 minutes.
4. In a small bowl, whisk together the eggs and salt. Add to the skillet and cook, scrambling, until the eggs are set, about 3 minutes. Remove from the heat and set aside.
5. In a blender or food processor, combine the tomatoes, roasted red peppers, and garlic. Blend on high until smooth.
6. Place the English muffins cut-side up on the prepared baking sheet.
7. Spread the muffins with the tomato-and-red-pepper sauce, and top with the egg mixture. Sprinkle with the cheese.
8. Bake until the cheese melts and begins to brown, about 10 minutes. Let cool slightly before serving.

Nutritional boost: **Make this heart-healthier by using 8 egg whites in place of the 4 whole eggs.**

Per Serving: Calories: 325; Total fat: 13g; Saturated fat: 4g; Cholesterol: 212mg; Carbohydrates: 30g; Fiber: 2g; Protein: 20g; Sodium: 895mg

PARMESAN ASPARAGUS MINI FRITTATAS

GLUTEN-FREE, VEGETARIAN

Serves 6 | Prep time: 5 minutes | Cook time: 15 minutes | Serving size: 2 frittatas

Not only are these little, pillowy bites of egg, cheese, and asparagus easy to make; they also freeze well and have a divine flavor from the herbs and spices in the eggs. If you do freeze them, reheat them in the microwave for a minute or two, and you'll have a quick and easy breakfast for those busy mornings.

Nonstick cooking spray

10 eggs

1 tablespoon skim milk

1 teaspoon Dijon mustard

½ teaspoon sea salt

½ teaspoon garlic powder

¼ teaspoon freshly ground black pepper

1 teaspoon dried Italian seasoning

5 asparagus spears, trimmed and cut into ½-inch pieces

½ cup shredded Parmesan cheese

1. Preheat the oven to 400°F. Spray a 12-cup muffin tin with nonstick cooking spray and set aside.
2. In a large bowl, whisk together the eggs, milk, mustard, salt, garlic powder, pepper, and Italian seasoning until well blended.
3. Fold in the asparagus and Parmesan cheese.
4. Spoon the mixture into the cups of the prepared muffin tin.
5. Bake until the eggs are set, about 15 minutes. Let cool slightly before serving.

Nutritional boost: Make this heart-healthier by reducing the whole eggs to 5, adding 10 egg whites, and omitting the Parmesan cheese or substituting a low-fat cheese, such as low-fat mozzarella.

Per Serving: Calories: 160; Total fat: 10g; Saturated fat: 4g; Cholesterol: 317mg; Carbohydrates: 2g; Fiber: <1g; Protein: 14g; Sodium: 460mg

QUICK AND EASY SHAKSHUKA

GLUTEN-FREE, VEGETARIAN

Serves 4 | Prep time: 10 minutes | Cook time: 25 minutes | Serving size: 1 egg and ¾ cup sauce

What happens when you cook your eggs in a savory, fragrant, spiced tomato sauce? Shakshuka! This belly-warming Mediterranean-inspired breakfast of poached eggs contains plenty of nutritious, heart-loving ingredients, perfect for a leisurely morning in.

2 tablespoons extra-virgin olive oil

1 onion, finely chopped

1 red bell pepper, seeded and finely chopped

2 garlic cloves, minced

1 (28-ounce) can crushed tomatoes

½ teaspoon paprika

1 teaspoon ground cumin

¼ teaspoon red pepper flakes

½ teaspoon sea salt

¼ teaspoon freshly ground black pepper

4 eggs

¼ cup chopped fresh cilantro

1. Preheat the oven to 375°F.
2. In a large ovenproof skillet, heat the olive oil over medium-high heat until it shimmers.
3. Add the onion and bell pepper and cook, stirring occasionally, until the vegetables soften, about 4 minutes.
4. Add the garlic and cook, stirring constantly, for 30 seconds.
5. Add the tomatoes with their juices, paprika, cumin, red pepper flakes, salt, and black pepper. Cook, stirring occasionally, until it boils. Reduce the heat to medium and simmer, stirring occasionally, for 5 minutes.
6. Using a wooden spoon, make four wells in the tomato sauce. Carefully crack an egg into each well.
7. Bake until the eggs are set, 10 to 12 minutes.
8. Sprinkle with the cilantro before serving.

Per Serving: Calories: 232; Total fat: 12g; Saturated fat: 3g; Cholesterol: 186mg; Carbohydrates: 21g; Fiber: 4g; Protein: 10g; Sodium: 936mg

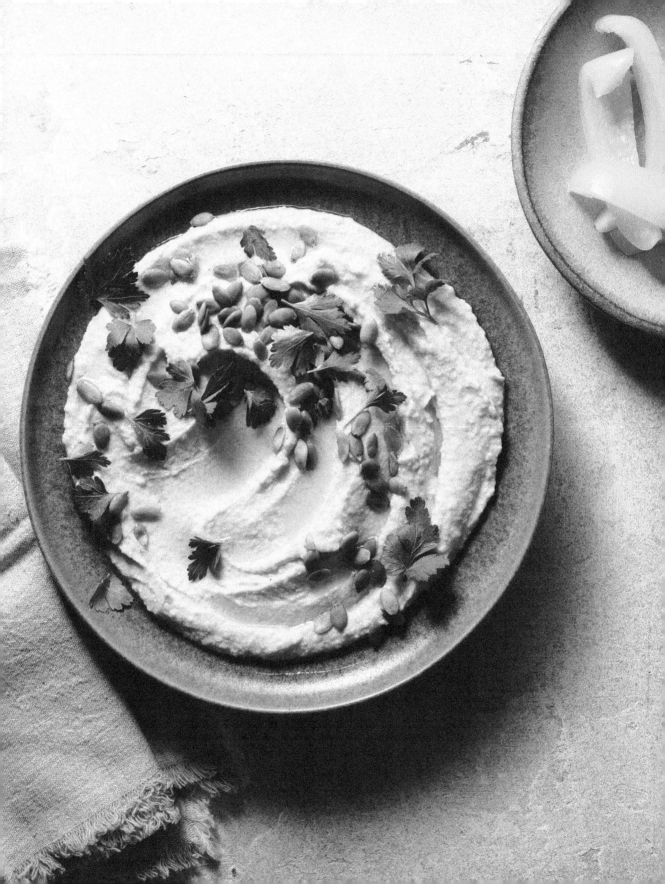

MEZZE DISHES

*< Easy Hummus,
page 32*

MARINATED OLIVES

ALLERGEN-FREE, GLUTEN-FREE, VEGAN

Serves 4 | Prep time: 10 minutes, plus 1 week to marinate | Cook time: 10 minutes | Serving size: ½ cup

These tiny fruits (yes, olives are a fruit!) are a staple in the Mediterranean diet. Rich in monounsaturated fats, olives have been linked to lowering inflammation and reducing heart disease. Sure, you can buy marinated olives, buy why not mix up your own briny marinade? To soak up all the delicious flavors, let the olives sit in the fridge for about a week.

2 cups olives (a good mix of types), rinsed

1 cup extra-virgin olive oil

Zest and juice of ½ orange

2 garlic cloves, sliced

¼ teaspoon red pepper flakes

1 tablespoon dried Italian seasoning

2 rosemary sprigs

1 tablespoon red wine vinegar

¼ teaspoon freshly ground black pepper

Juice of 1 lemon

1. Put the olives in a nonreactive sealable container, such as a canning jar.
2. In a small saucepan over low heat, combine the olive oil, orange zest and juice, garlic, red pepper flakes, Italian seasoning, rosemary sprigs, red wine vinegar, and black pepper.
3. Cover and simmer, stirring occasionally, for 10 minutes.
4. Remove from the heat and stir in the lemon juice. Allow to cool.
5. Pour the marinade over the olives and seal. Refrigerate for at least 1 week. Enjoy.

Variation tip: If you prefer to use fresh herbs, you can replace the dried Italian seasoning with 2 thyme sprigs, 6 basil leaves, and 4 oregano sprigs. For spicier olives, add up to another ½ teaspoon of red pepper flakes. For milder olives, reduce the amount of red pepper flakes or omit them.

Per Serving: Calories: 565; Total fat: 62g; Saturated fat: 7g; Cholesterol: 0mg; Carbohydrates: 7g; Fiber: 1g; Protein: <1g; Sodium: 188mg

HUMMUS DEVILED EGGS WITH ROASTED RED PEPPERS

GLUTEN-FREE, VEGETARIAN

Serves 12 | Prep time: 10 minutes | Serving size: 2 egg halves

With a savory, creamy filling, these deviled eggs make the perfect small bite for your mezze platter. To save time, you can buy eggs already hard-boiled, or hard-boil them yourself in about 15 minutes. Make sure the eggs are completely cooled before you work with them.

12 hard-boiled eggs, halved lengthwise (see Ingredient tip on page 24)

¼ cup Easy Hummus (page 32) or store-bought hummus

2 tablespoons nonfat plain Greek yogurt

1 tablespoon red wine vinegar

2 teaspoons Dijon mustard

1 garlic clove, finely minced

½ teaspoon sea salt

¼ teaspoon freshly ground black pepper

½ (12-ounce) jar roasted red peppers, drained, patted dry, and finely chopped

4 basil leaves, finely chopped

2 tablespoons capers, drained and rinsed

1. Spoon the yolks out of the eggs and put them in a bowl. Place the whites, cut-side up, on a platter.
2. Mash the egg yolks with a fork until broken into very small pieces.
3. Add the hummus, yogurt, red wine vinegar, mustard, garlic, salt, and black pepper to the bowl. Stir until well combined.
4. Fold in the roasted red peppers until just combined.
5. Spoon or pipe the filling into the egg halves.
6. Garnish with the basil and capers before serving.

Substitution tip: Make this dairy-free by replacing the Greek yogurt with olive oil mayonnaise.

Per Serving: Calories: 97; Total fat: 6g; Saturated fat: 2g; Cholesterol: 186mg; Carbohydrates: 2g; Fiber: 1g; Protein: 7g; Sodium: 243mg

EASY HUMMUS

ALLERGEN-FREE, GLUTEN-FREE, VEGAN

Serves 8 | Prep time: 10 minutes | Serving size: ¼ cup hummus and ¼ red bell pepper

With lemony flavor and lots of spice, hummus makes the perfect dip. It pairs especially well with sweet, crunchy red bell peppers, but you can try other delicious veggies for dipping, such as jicama, sliced carrots, or sliced radishes. You'll enjoy this as a dip, a sandwich spread, or even in an omelet.

1 (15-ounce) can chickpeas, drained and rinsed

½ cup tahini

Juice of 2 lemons

1 garlic clove, minced

2 tablespoons extra-virgin olive oil, plus a drizzle for garnish

½ teaspoon sea salt

Water, as needed

¼ cup chopped fresh Italian parsley

2 red bell peppers, seeded and sliced, for serving

1. In a blender or food processor, combine the chickpeas, tahini, lemon juice, garlic, olive oil, and salt. Blend until smooth.
2. Check the consistency, and add water and blend to reach your desired texture.
3. Spoon into a bowl. Garnish with a drizzle of olive oil and the parsley.
4. Serve with the red bell peppers for dipping.

Nutritional boost: Garnish with a sprinkling of ¼ cup of pepitas to add crunch and heart-healthy antioxidants and fats to this tasty snack.

Per Serving: Calories: 140; Total fat: 8g; Saturated fat: 1g; Cholesterol: 0mg; Carbohydrates: 14g; Fiber: 4g; Protein: 4g; Sodium: 156mg

LEBANESE-SPICED ROASTED CHICKPEAS

ALLERGEN-FREE, GLUTEN-FREE, VEGAN

Serves 8 | Prep time: 10 minutes | Cook time: 30 minutes | Serving size: ¼ cup

This Mediterranean-inspired tasty, spicy snack is ideal for increasing fiber for heart health. The warm spices complement the crunch of the chickpeas, and the dish travels well, so this is the perfect on-the-go snack.

1 (15-ounce) can chickpeas, drained, rinsed, and patted dry

1 tablespoon extra-virgin olive oil

½ teaspoon sea salt

¼ teaspoon freshly ground black pepper

¼ teaspoon ground cumin

¼ teaspoon ground coriander

⅛ teaspoon ground cloves

1 teaspoon ground cinnamon

1. Preheat the oven to 400°F. Line a baking sheet with parchment paper and set aside.
2. In a bowl, combine the chickpeas, olive oil, salt, pepper, cumin, coriander, cloves, and cinnamon. Toss to mix well.
3. Spread the mixture in a thin layer on the prepared baking sheet.
4. Bake for 20 minutes. Remove from the oven, stir, and continue baking for an additional 10 minutes.
5. Turn the oven off and allow the chickpeas to cool completely in the oven before serving.

Per Serving: Calories: 69; Total fat: 2g; Saturated fat: <1g; Cholesterol: 0mg; Carbohydrates: 10g; Fiber: 3g; Protein: 3g; Sodium: 146mg

SHRIMP CEVICHE

GLUTEN-FREE

Serves 4 | Prep time: 10 minutes, plus 30 minutes to chill | Serving size: ½ cup

While ceviche typically uses raw seafood and allows the acids in the citrus to "cook" it, this version uses cooked bay shrimp, which are easily available fresh or frozen in most grocery stores. With a little acid, a little spice, and lots of sweet, fresh flavor from the citrus and shrimp, this is a truly delicious and easy mezze dish.

1 pound cooked baby shrimp, drained and rinsed

Juice of 1 lime

Juice of 1 lemon

Juice of ½ orange

1 tablespoon extra-virgin olive oil

1 tomato, seeded and chopped

½ red onion, minced

1 red chile, seeded and minced

2 tablespoons chopped fresh cilantro

½ teaspoon sea salt

1. In a medium bowl, combine the shrimp, lime juice, lemon juice, orange juice, olive oil, tomato, onion, chile, cilantro, and salt. Stir well.
2. Allow to rest in the fridge, covered, for 30 minutes before serving.

Substitution tip: If you're allergic to shellfish but not fish, you can replace the shrimp with chopped cooked halibut, salmon, or cod.

Per Serving: Calories: 170; Total fat: 5g; Saturated fat: 1g; Cholesterol: 220mg; Carbohydrates: 4g; Fiber: 1g; Protein: 24g; Sodium: 550mg

BAKED PARMESAN ZUCCHINI STRIPS

GLUTEN-FREE, VEGETARIAN

Serves 4 | Prep time: 10 minutes | Cook time: 35 minutes | Serving size: 8 strips

Tender zucchini with herbs and Parmesan cheese? It's a delicious snack and a tasty side dish that's sure to delight even the most finicky vegetable avoider. Serve these hot and fresh from the oven either alone or with some marinara sauce for dipping.

½ cup grated
Parmesan cheese

1 tablespoon dried Italian
seasoning

¼ teaspoon garlic powder

½ teaspoon sea salt

Pinch red pepper flakes

4 small zucchini, quartered
lengthwise and each
quarter halved

2 tablespoons extra-virgin
olive oil

1. Preheat the oven to 350°F. Line a baking sheet with parchment paper and set aside.

2. In a small bowl, combine the Parmesan cheese, Italian seasoning, garlic powder, salt, and red pepper flakes.

3. In a large bowl, combine the zucchini strips with the olive oil and toss to coat. Add the spice blend and toss to coat again.

4. Spread the zucchini strips in a single layer on the prepared baking sheet. Bake until the zucchini is tender, about 30 minutes.

5. Turn the oven to broil. Broil for 3 minutes to crisp the coating. Let cool slightly before serving.

Variation tip: This recipe works with any summer squash, including yellow or pattypan squash.

Per Serving: Calories: 140; Total fat: 11g; Saturated fat: 4g; Cholesterol: 10mg; Carbohydrates: 5g; Fiber: 2g; Protein: 7g; Sodium: 536mg

MEDITERRANEAN-SPICED SALSA WITH PITA CHIPS

VEGAN

Serves 4 | Prep time: 10 minutes | Cook time: 15 minutes | Serving size: ¼ cup salsa and 8 pita chips

Crisp pita chips are a delicious, crunchy alternative to traditional tortilla chips. They take a few minutes to bake, but with a nontraditional Mediterranean-spiced salsa for dipping, the result is delicious. You can make both ahead of time and refrigerate the salsa for up to three days. Keep the chips in an airtight container at room temperature.

4 whole-wheat pitas, each cut into 8 wedges

4 tablespoons extra-virgin olive oil, divided

¾ teaspoon sea salt, divided

½ cup Marinated Olives (page 30), pitted and chopped

2 tomatoes, seeded and chopped

¼ red onion, finely chopped

½ (12-ounce) jar roasted red peppers, drained and chopped

2 garlic cloves, finely minced

Zest of ½ lemon and juice of 1 lemon

2 tablespoons chopped fresh Italian parsley

1. Preheat the oven to 375°F. Line a baking sheet with parchment paper.
2. Brush the pita wedges with 2 tablespoons of olive oil. Spread them in a single layer on the prepared baking sheet and sprinkle with ¼ teaspoon of salt.
3. Bake until crisp, 12 to 15 minutes. Cool.
4. While the chips cool, in a medium bowl, combine the olives, tomatoes, red onion, roasted red peppers, garlic, lemon zest and juice, remaining 2 tablespoons of oil, remaining ½ teaspoon of salt, and the parsley.
5. Serve the cooled chips with the salsa.

Substitution tip: If you have a gluten intolerance or celiac disease, replace the pita chips with sliced jicama or gluten-free whole-grain crackers for dipping.

Per Serving: Calories: 436; Total fat: 32g; Saturated fat: 4g; Cholesterol: 0mg; Carbohydrates: 37g; Fiber: 6g; Protein: 7g; Sodium: 641mg

CUMIN ROASTED ROOT VEGETABLES

ALLERGY-FREE, GLUTEN-FREE, VEGAN

Serves 4 | Prep time: 10 minutes | Cook time: 45 minutes | Serving size: 1 cup

Antioxidant- and fiber-rich roasted root vegetables are delicious in a mezze platter or as a simple and deeply flavorful side dish. Roasting brings out deep, caramelized flavors in the vegetables and enhances this dish's satisfying savory notes.

4 beets, scrubbed, trimmed, and quartered lengthwise

4 carrots, peeled and cut into sticks

6 shallots, peeled and quartered lengthwise

1 sweet potato, peeled and cut into sticks

2 tablespoons extra-virgin olive oil

1 teaspoon ground cumin

½ teaspoon garlic powder

½ teaspoon sea salt

¼ teaspoon freshly ground black pepper

1. Preheat the oven to 425°F. Line two baking sheets with parchment paper and set aside.

2. In a large bowl, combine the beets, carrots, shallots, sweet potato, olive oil, cumin, garlic powder, salt, and pepper. Toss to mix.

3. Spread in a single layer on the prepared baking sheets.

4. Bake until the vegetables are tender and browned, about 45 minutes. Let cool slightly before serving.

Per Serving: Calories: 180; Total fat: 8g; Saturated fat: 1g; Cholesterol: 0mg; Carbohydrates: 27g; Fiber: 5g; Protein: 3g; Sodium: 406mg

MOROCCAN-SPICED TURKEY MEATBALLS

ALLERGEN-FREE, GLUTEN-FREE

Serves 4 | Prep time: 10 minutes | Cook time: 25 minutes | Serving size: 5 or 6 meatballs

These turkey meatballs are so fragrant! They smell amazing when they cook. And with warm spices, they taste pretty darn good. These are delicious as an appetizer or snack, and they're absolutely perfect in sandwiches, too.

2 tablespoons extra-virgin olive oil

½ red onion, finely minced

3 garlic cloves, minced

1 pound ground turkey breast

2 tablespoons chopped fresh mint

2 tablespoons chopped fresh Italian parsley

½ teaspoon ground coriander

½ teaspoon ground cinnamon

½ teaspoon ground cumin

½ teaspoon sea salt

¼ teaspoon freshly ground black pepper

1 egg, beaten

1. Preheat the oven to 400°F. Line a rimmed baking sheet with parchment paper and set aside.
2. In a medium skillet, heat the olive oil over medium-high heat until it shimmers.
3. Add the onion and cook until soft, about 3 minutes.
4. Add the garlic and cook, stirring constantly, for 30 seconds. Remove the skillet from the heat and let cool.
5. In a large bowl, combine the turkey, mint, parsley, coriander, cinnamon, cumin, salt, pepper, and egg. Add the cooled onion and garlic. Mix well.
6. Form the mixture into 1-inch balls and place them on the prepared baking sheet.
7. Bake until the meatballs are browned and reach an internal temperature of 165°F, about 20 minutes. Let cool slightly before serving.

Per Serving: Calories: 210; Total fat: 10g; Saturated fat: 2g; Cholesterol: 102mg; Carbohydrates: 3g; Fiber: 1g; Protein: 28g; Sodium: 382mg

MEZZE PLATTER

Serves 12 to 15 | **Prep time: 10 minutes** | **Serving size: A small sample of each component**

There's no need to compromise your health needs when you attend or throw a party. Instead, put together a tasty mezze platter. Then you'll be sure you have something to eat that's delicious and supports your heart health.

1 recipe Marinated Olives (page 30)

2 cucumbers, sliced

1 recipe Easy Hummus (page 32)

1 pint cherry tomatoes

1 recipe White Bean Dip (page 66)

1 recipe Mediterranean-Spiced Salsa with Pita Chips (page 36)

1 (6.5-ounce) jar marinated artichoke hearts, drained

1 (12-ounce) jar roasted red peppers, drained

1 cup almonds

1 recipe Tabbouleh (page 42)

Multigrain crackers

Place the olives, cucumbers, hummus, tomatoes, white bean dip, salsa with pita chips, artichoke hearts, roasted red peppers, almonds, tabbouleh, and crackers in a satisfying arrangement on a wooden cheese plate or a large platter. Serve.

Substitution tip: It's easy to customize this platter for people with various allergies by changing ingredients. You can use any of the cold foods in this chapter, salads in chapter 4, spreads in chapter 5, chopped fresh vegetables, and whole-wheat pita bread. If making it gluten-free, opt for gluten-free crackers and omit the tabbouleh. For nut allergies, omit the almonds.

Per Serving: Calories: 718; Total fat: 53g; Saturated fat: 6g; Cholesterol: 0mg; Carbohydrates: 55g; Fiber: 14g; Protein: 15g; Sodium: 843mg

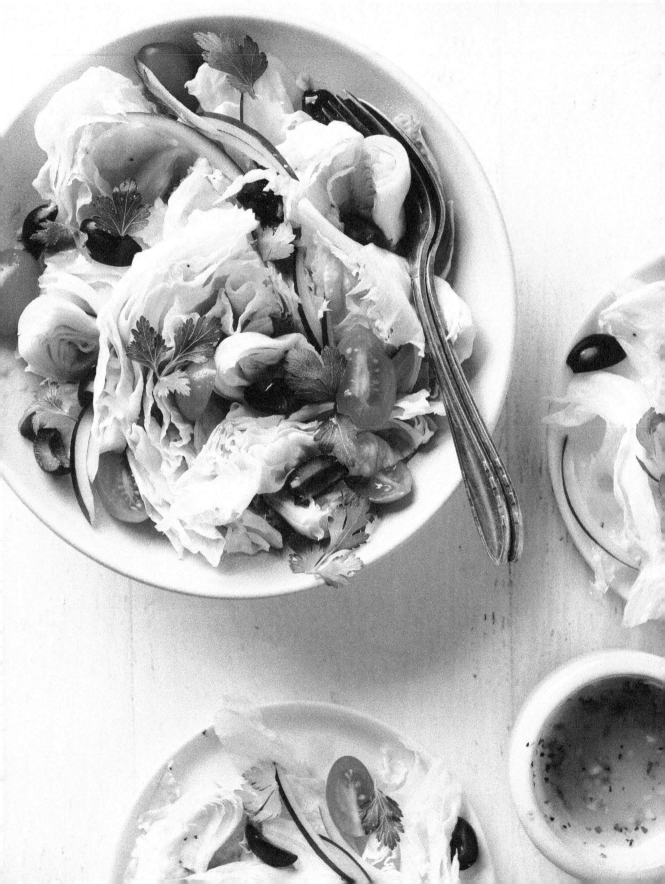

— CHAPTER 4 —

SOUPS AND SALADS

< *Easy Greek Salad,*
page 46

TABBOULEH

VEGAN

Serves 4 | Prep time: 30 minutes | Serving size: ¾ cup

Tabbouleh is a feast for the senses. This brightly colored, heart-healthy Mediterranean-inspired bulgur wheat salad is beautiful, aromatic, and redolent with the flavor of fresh herbs and vegetables. It's equally delicious as a lunch main, added to a mezze platter, or as a side dish for a lovely piece of fish or poultry.

2 tomatoes, diced

2 cucumbers, diced

¾ teaspoon sea salt, divided

1 bunch scallions,
    thinly sliced

2 bunches fresh parsley,
    stemmed and
    finely chopped

1 bunch fresh mint, stemmed
    and finely chopped

⅔ cup bulgur, cooked
    according to package
    directions and cooled
    (2 cups cooked)

Juice of 2 lemons

¼ cup extra-virgin olive oil

1 garlic clove, minced

½ teaspoon Dijon mustard

1. Put the tomatoes and cucumbers in a colander over a bowl or in the sink and salt them with ½ teaspoon of salt. Allow to sit to drain the juices for 15 minutes.

2. In a large bowl, combine the drained tomatoes and cucumbers, scallions, parsley, mint, and bulgur. Stir well.

3. In a small bowl, whisk together the lemon juice, olive oil, garlic, mustard, and remaining ¼ teaspoon of salt to make the dressing.

4. Toss the salad with the dressing. Let sit for 10 minutes to allow the flavors to blend before serving.

Substitution tip: You can make this gluten-free by replacing the bulgur with 2 cups of cooked brown rice or 2 cups of cooked quinoa.

Per Serving: Calories: 270; Total fat: 15g; Saturated fat: 2g; Cholesterol: 0mg; Carbohydrates: 33g; Fiber: 9g; Protein: 7g; Sodium: 506mg

QUINOA SALAD

ALLERGEN-FREE, GLUTEN-FREE, VEGAN

Serves 4 | Prep time: 20 minutes | Cook time: 15 minutes | Serving size: 1 cup

Quinoa is a delicious, gluten-free food containing fats that help boost "good" cholesterol. This colorful, sweet, and savory salad with roasted red peppers, red onion, and Spanish olives pairs beautifully with a fragrant and flavorful vinaigrette.

1¼ water

1 cup uncooked quinoa

1 cup Spanish olives, pitted and halved

1 (12-ounce) jar roasted red peppers, drained and chopped

½ red onion, minced

¼ cup chopped fresh Italian parsley

3 tablespoons red wine vinegar

¼ cup extra-virgin olive oil

½ teaspoon Dijon mustard

½ teaspoon smoked paprika

2 garlic cloves, minced

½ teaspoon sea salt

1. In a small pan, bring the water to a boil and add the quinoa. Reduce the heat to low and simmer for 10 to 15 minutes, covered, until the quinoa is soft. Fluff with a fork and allow the quinoa to cool before proceeding.

2. In a large bowl, combine the cooked quinoa, olives, roasted red peppers, onion, and parsley.

3. In a small bowl, whisk together the red wine vinegar, olive oil, mustard, paprika, garlic, and salt to make the dressing.

4. Toss the salad with the dressing. Let sit for 10 minutes to allow the flavors to blend before serving.

Nutritional boost: Add 1 cup of flaked cooked salmon or drained albacore tuna to add protein and heart-healthy fats.

Per Serving: Calories: 371; Total fat: 20g; Saturated fat: 3g; Cholesterol: 0mg; Carbohydrates: 39g; Fiber: 5g; Protein: 7g; Sodium: 686mg

LEMON-CUCUMBER SALAD

GLUTEN-FREE, VEGETARIAN

Serves 4 | Prep time: 15 minutes | Serving size: 1½ cups

With a bright, garlicky lemon dressing, crunchy cucumbers, tangy tomatoes, and salty feta cheese, this quick salad is the perfect mix of flavors, textures, and colors.

2 medium
  cucumbers, chopped

2 pints grape
  tomatoes, halved

½ red onion, finely chopped

¼ cup chopped fresh parsley

¼ cup chopped fresh mint

½ cup crumbled feta cheese

Juice of 1½ lemons

¼ cup extra-virgin olive oil

3 garlic cloves, minced

½ teaspoon Dijon mustard

½ teaspoon sea salt

1. In a large bowl, combine the cucumbers, tomatoes, red onion, parsley, mint, and feta cheese.
2. In a small bowl, whisk together the lemon juice, olive oil, garlic, mustard, and salt to make the dressing.
3. Toss the salad with the dressing and serve immediately.

Per Serving: Calories: 236; Total fat: 18g; Saturated fat: 5g; Cholesterol: 17mg; Carbohydrates: 16g; Fiber: 4g; Protein: 6g; Sodium: 536mg

ITALIAN-STYLE CHOPPED SALAD

GLUTEN-FREE, VEGAN

Serves 4 | Prep time: 15 minutes | Serving size: 2½ cups

There's something so satisfying about a chopped salad. The nice variety of different veggies adds a ton of texture. Easily turn this into a main dish by adding a protein, such as chopped fish, poultry, or even marinated tofu.

1 pint grape
tomatoes, halved

1 red onion, finely chopped

1 (14-ounce) can
artichoke hearts or
bottoms, chopped

½ cup olives, pitted
and chopped

1 head iceberg
lettuce, chopped

¼ cup chopped fresh
Italian parsley

3 tablespoons red
wine vinegar

¼ cup extra-virgin olive oil

2 garlic cloves, minced

1 teaspoon dried Italian
seasoning

½ teaspoon Dijon mustard

½ teaspoon sea salt

¼ teaspoon freshly ground
black pepper

Pinch red pepper flakes

1. In a large bowl, combine the tomatoes, red onion, artichoke hearts, olives, lettuce, and parsley.

2. In a small bowl, whisk together the red wine vinegar, olive oil, garlic, Italian seasoning, mustard, salt, black pepper, and red pepper flakes to make the dressing.

3. Toss the salad with the dressing and serve immediately.

Nutritional boost: Boost heart health by adding ¼ cup of pine nuts or pepitas to the salad. Pine nuts are loaded with heart-healthy ingredients, and they would add an enticing crunch to this salad.

Per Serving: Calories: 223; Total fat: 16g; Saturated fat: 2g; Cholesterol: 0mg; Carbohydrates: 17g; Fiber: 6g; Protein: 4g; Sodium: 772mg

EASY GREEK SALAD

GLUTEN-FREE, VEGETARIAN

Serves 4 | Prep time: 15 minutes | Serving size: 1½ cups

Greek salads are beautifully fresh and colorful, and they're packed with delicious flavors and textures. This simple Greek salad doesn't take long to prepare, and it's a tasty and nutritional cardiovascular powerhouse, making it the perfect side dish.

1 cucumber, halved lengthwise, seeded, and sliced

1 red onion, quartered and cut into thin slices

1 pint cherry tomatoes

1 cup black olives, pitted and halved

½ cup crumbled feta cheese

3 tablespoons red wine vinegar

¼ cup extra-virgin olive oil

3 garlic cloves, minced

1 tablespoon dried oregano

½ teaspoon sea salt

¼ teaspoon freshly ground black pepper

1. In a large bowl, combine the cucumber, onion, tomatoes, olives, and feta cheese.
2. In a small bowl, whisk together the red wine vinegar, olive oil, garlic, oregano, salt, and pepper to make the dressing.
3. Toss the salad with the dressing and serve immediately.

Substitution tip: You can make this vegan-friendly and dairy-free by omitting the feta cheese altogether or by substituting vegan feta cheese.

Per Serving: Calories: 250; Total fat: 22g; Saturated fat: 5g; Cholesterol: 17mg; Carbohydrates: 12g; Fiber: 4g; Protein: 5g; Sodium: 803mg

BALELA SALAD

ALLERGEN-FREE, GLUTEN-FREE, VEGAN

Serves 4 | Prep time: 30 minutes | Serving size: 1½ cups

Here's the ideal salad. Featuring creamy beans, fresh herbs, and bright flavors, this meal provides an excellent source of fiber, protein, and B vitamins, helping improve cholesterol levels while maintaining good gut health.

2 (15-ounce) can chickpeas, drained and rinsed

1 pint cherry tomatoes, halved

1 bunch scallions, thinly sliced

½ cup pitted black olives, halved

½ (8-ounce) jar sun-dried tomatoes, drained and chopped

½ cup basil leaves, chopped

2 tablespoons red wine vinegar

Zest and juice of 1 lemon

¼ cup extra-virgin olive oil

2 garlic cloves, minced

½ teaspoon paprika

½ teaspoon sea salt

1. In a large bowl, combine the chickpeas, cherry tomatoes, scallions, olives, sun-dried tomatoes, and basil.

2. In a small bowl, whisk together the red wine vinegar, lemon zest and juice, olive oil, garlic, paprika, and salt to make the dressing.

3. Toss the salad with dressing. Allow to rest for 15 minutes to let the flavors blend before serving.

Per Serving: Calories: 411; Total fat: 20g; Saturated fat: 2g; Cholesterol: 0mg; Carbohydrates: 50g; Fiber: 14g; Protein: 12g; Sodium: 449mg

FRAGRANT TOMATO AND HERB SALAD

ALLERGEN-FREE, GLUTEN-FREE, VEGAN

Serves 4 | Prep time: 15 minutes | Serving size: 1¾ cups

Garden-fresh seasonal tomatoes have the perfect amount of sweetness and acidity for this special salad. Better yet, tomatoes are rich sources of lycopene and potassium, which are key nutrients for lowering "bad" cholesterol to prevent blood clotting.

6 cups chopped heirloom or cherry tomatoes

¼ cup chopped fresh Italian parsley

¼ cup chopped fresh basil leaves

¼ cup chopped fresh dill

¼ cup chopped fresh mint

3 tablespoons balsamic vinegar

¼ cup extra-virgin olive oil

½ teaspoon sea salt

½ teaspoon freshly ground black pepper

1. In a large bowl, combine the tomatoes, parsley, basil, dill, and mint.
2. In a small bowl, whisk together the balsamic vinegar, olive oil, salt, and pepper to make the dressing.
3. Toss the salad with the dressing and serve immediately.

Nutritional boost: Add texture and heart-healthy fats by adding ¼ cup of finely chopped almonds.

Per Serving: Calories: 178; Total fat: 14g; Saturated fat: 2g; Cholesterol: 0mg; Carbohydrates: 13g; Fiber: 3g; Protein: 2g; Sodium: 323mg

POTATO SALAD WITH GREEK YOGURT AND HERB DRESSING

GLUTEN-FREE, VEGETARIAN

Serves 6 | Prep time: 10 minutes, plus 2 hours to chill | Cook time: 15 minutes | Serving size: 1½ cups

Yes, potatoes can be part of a heart-healthy diet. As long as they are not deep-fried, their potassium, vitamin C, and fiber are good for your heart. And when mixed with herbs and Greek yogurt, it's a tantalizing experience for your taste buds.

3 pounds baby red potatoes, quartered

½ red onion, finely chopped

1 cup fresh or frozen peas, cooked and drained

1½ cups nonfat plain Greek yogurt

1 teaspoon Dijon mustard

1 tablespoon red wine vinegar

¼ cup chopped fresh dill

½ cup chopped fresh Italian parsley

10 basil leaves, finely chopped

½ teaspoon sea salt

¼ teaspoon freshly ground black pepper

1. In a large pot, cover the potatoes with water, and bring to a boil over high heat. Cover and cook until the potatoes are fork-tender, about 15 minutes. Run the potatoes under cold water to stop the cooking. Drain thoroughly, pat dry, and let cool.

2. Put the cooled potatoes in a large bowl, then add the red onion and peas.

3. In a small bowl, whisk together the yogurt, mustard, red wine vinegar, dill, parsley, basil, salt, and pepper to make the dressing.

4. Toss the potatoes with the dressing. Chill for 2 hours before serving.

Substitution tip: You can make this vegan and dairy-free by using a nondairy plain yogurt in place of the Greek yogurt or by substituting it with 1 cup of nondairy yogurt and ½ cup of vegan mayonnaise.

Per Serving: Calories: 217; Total fat: <1g; Saturated fat: 0g; Cholesterol: 0mg; Carbohydrates: 43g; Fiber: 5g; Protein: 11g; Sodium: 309mg

PASTA SALAD WITH BROCCOLI AND TOMATOES

VEGETARIAN

Serves 6 | Prep time: 10 minutes, plus 2 hours to chill | Serving size: 1½ cups

With plenty of colors and flavors, this salad is savory and yummy. It has great Italian herbs that pair well with the crunch of fresh broccoli and the toothsome bite of pasta. Sun-dried tomatoes add just a hint of sweetness.

8 ounces whole-wheat farfalle (bowtie) pasta, cooked according to package directions, drained, and cooled

½ red onion, finely chopped

1 red bell pepper, seeded and chopped

2 cups broccoli florets, cut into small pieces

½ (8-ounce) jar sun-dried tomatoes, drained

1 pint grape tomatoes, halved

¼ cup chopped fresh basil

¼ cup pepitas

½ cup nonfat plain Greek yogurt

2 tablespoons red wine vinegar

2 garlic cloves, minced

½ teaspoon sea salt

1. In a large bowl, combine the pasta, onion, bell pepper, broccoli, sun-dried tomatoes, grape tomatoes, basil, and pepitas.
2. In a small bowl, whisk together the yogurt, red wine vinegar, garlic, and salt to make the dressing.
3. Toss the salad with the dressing. Chill for 2 hours before serving.

Substitution tip: You can make this gluten-free by replacing the whole-wheat farfalle with a gluten-free farfalle or any gluten-free pasta in a short shape, such as rotini or penne.

Per Serving: Calories: 222; Total fat: 5g; Saturated fat: 1g; Cholesterol: 0mg; Carbohydrates: 32g; Fiber: 7g; Protein: 11g; Sodium: 241mg

ARTICHOKE AND OLIVE SALAD

ALLERGEN-FREE, GLUTEN-FREE, VEGAN

Serves 4 | Prep time: 10 minutes, plus 2 hours to chill | Serving size: 1 cup

A bright lemon dressing and fresh herbs bring this simple salad to life. You can find artichoke bottoms in the canned-vegetable aisle; they're already cooked and ready to add straight to this delicious salad.

2 (15-ounce) cans artichoke bottoms, drained and chopped

1 cup Spanish olives, pitted and chopped

1 red bell pepper, seeded and chopped

1 pint cherry tomatoes, halved

¼ cup chopped fresh basil

¼ cup chopped fresh dill

¼ cup extra-virgin olive oil

3 tablespoons red wine vinegar

1 garlic clove, minced

½ teaspoon Dijon mustard

1 teaspoon dried Italian seasoning

½ teaspoon sea salt

1. In a large bowl, combine the artichoke bottoms, olives, bell pepper, tomatoes, basil, and dill.

2. In a small bowl, whisk together the olive oil, red wine vinegar, garlic, mustard, Italian seasoning, and salt to make the dressing.

3. Toss the salad with the dressing. Chill for 2 hours before serving.

Per Serving: Calories: 174; Total fat: 12g; Saturated fat: 2g; Cholesterol: 0mg; Carbohydrates: 13g; Fiber: 6g; Protein: 3g; Sodium: 682mg

SWEET POTATO AND LEEK SOUP

GLUTEN-FREE, VEGETARIAN

Serves 4 | Prep time: 10 minutes | Cook time: 20 minutes | Serving size: 1½ cups

Potato-leek soup is a classic, but this recipe adds intriguing Mediterranean flavors along with the earthy sweetness of sweet potatoes rich with potassium and magnesium, which help regulate blood pressure. Be sure to make a double batch to freeze for busy days when you have little time to cook.

2 tablespoons extra-virgin olive oil, plus a drizzle for garnish

3 leeks, chopped and rinsed (see Ingredient tip)

2 teaspoons ground cumin

½ teaspoon ground allspice

½ teaspoon sea salt

3 garlic cloves, minced

4 cups low-sodium vegetable broth

3 sweet potatoes, peeled and cut into ½-inch dice

½ cup skim milk or nondairy milk

¼ cup pepitas

1. In a large pot, heat the olive oil over medium-high heat until it shimmers.
2. Add the leeks, cumin, allspice, and salt. Cook, stirring occasionally, until the leeks are tender, about 4 minutes.
3. Add the garlic and cook, stirring constantly, for 30 seconds.
4. Add the broth and sweet potatoes. Bring to a boil.
5. Reduce the heat to medium-low. Simmer, stirring occasionally, until the potatoes are tender, 10 to 15 minutes.
6. Transfer the hot soup to a blender or food processor and add the milk. Fold a clean dish towel in quarters and place it on top of the blender or food processor lid. Put your hand on top of the towel to hold the lid in place and protect your hand from heat and burns. Blend or process on high for 30 seconds. Carefully vent the steam by lifting the lid away from your body and face. Blend until smooth, venting the steam every 30 to 60 seconds.
7. Serve garnished with a drizzle of extra-virgin olive oil and pepitas.

Ingredient tip: Leeks have lots of dirt trapped in between their layers. In order to wash them thoroughly, cut off the root end and the tough part at the top of the greens. You'll have some white part and some tender green part left. Quarter each leek lengthwise, cut into small pieces, and put in a large bowl of cold water. Agitate the leek pieces in the water with your fingers and allow the dirt to settle. Pour off the water and dirt, add more water, and repeat the process until no dirt settles in the bottom of the bowl. Pat the leeks dry with a paper towel before cooking them.

Per Serving: Calories: 281; Total fat: 12g; Saturated fat: 2g; Cholesterol: 1mg; Carbohydrates: 39; Fiber: 6g; Protein: 7g; Sodium: 498mg

MINESTRONE

VEGAN

Serves 6 | Prep time: 10 minutes | Cook time: 20 minutes | Serving size: 2 cups

This classic Italian vegetable soup is loaded with tender, antioxidant-rich veggies. If you're a fan of the flavor profile of tomatoes, herbs, and garlic, you'll love this soup. It also freezes well for up to six months.

2 tablespoons extra-virgin olive oil

1 onion, finely chopped

3 carrots, peeled and chopped

1 fennel bulb, chopped

4 garlic cloves, minced

4 cups low-sodium vegetable broth

1 (15-ounce) can low-sodium kidney beans, drained and rinsed

1 (15-ounce) can crushed tomatoes

1 small zucchini, chopped

2 cups chopped green beans

1 tablespoon dried Italian seasoning

½ teaspoon sea salt

1 cup elbow macaroni

1. In a large pot, heat the olive oil over medium-high heat until it shimmers.
2. Add the onion, carrots, and fennel. Cook, stirring occasionally, until the vegetables soften, about 5 minutes.
3. Add the garlic and cook, stirring constantly, for 30 seconds.
4. Add the broth, kidney beans, tomatoes with their juices, zucchini, green beans, Italian seasoning, and salt. Bring to a boil.
5. Add the elbow macaroni. Bring back to a boil. Reduce the heat to medium and cook, stirring occasionally, until the pasta is al dente, about 10 minutes. Serve.

Substitution tip: To make this gluten-free, you can use gluten-free pasta or omit the pasta altogether.

Per Serving: Calories: 248; Total fat: 6g; Saturated fat: 1g; Cholesterol: 0mg; Carbohydrates: 41g; Fiber: 10g; Protein: 11g; Sodium: 492mg

PASTA E FAGIOLI SOUP

Serves 6 | Prep time: 10 minutes | Cook time: 20 minutes | Serving size: 2 cups

This *zuppa Italiano* (Italian soup) is a favorite, and it's easy to see why. With creamy white beans, flavorful greens, aromatic turkey sausage, and tender vegetables, it's packed with yummy flavors and aromas.

2 tablespoons extra-virgin olive oil

1 pound Italian turkey sausage

1 onion, chopped

2 carrots, peeled and chopped

4 garlic cloves, minced

3 cups low-sodium chicken broth

2 cups chopped kale

1 (15-ounce) can white beans, drained and rinsed

2 (15-ounce) cans crushed tomatoes

1 tablespoon dried Italian seasoning

½ teaspoon sea salt

1 cup whole-wheat ditalini or tubettini pasta

1. In a large pot, heat the olive oil over medium-high heat until it shimmers. Add the Italian turkey sausage and cook, crumbling with a spoon, until it is browned, about 5 minutes. Using a slotted spoon, remove the sausage from the rendered fat in the pot and set it aside.

2. In the same pot, add the onion and carrots to the rendered fat. Cook, stirring occasionally, until the vegetables are soft, about 5 minutes.

3. Add the garlic and cook, stirring constantly, for 30 seconds.

4. Add the broth, kale, white beans, tomatoes with their juices, Italian seasoning, and salt. Bring to a boil.

5. Add the pasta and bring back to a boil. Reduce the heat to medium. Cook, stirring occasionally, until the pasta is al dente, about 6 minutes.

6. Return the sausage to the pot. Cook, stirring, until the sausage is heated through again, 1 to 2 minutes longer. Serve.

Ingredient tip: To add even more savory flavor, cut the rind from a wedge of Parmigiano-Reggiano cheese and add it to the pot when you add the broth. Remove what's left of the rind before serving.

Per Serving: Calories: 371; Total fat: 14g; Saturated fat: 3g; Cholesterol: 50mg; Carbohydrates: 37g; Fiber: 8g; Protein: 28g; Sodium: 1,058mg

WHITE BEAN SOUP WITH KALE AND SWEET POTATO

ALLERGEN-FREE, GLUTEN-FREE, VEGAN

Serves 6 | Prep time: 10 minutes | Cook time: 20 minutes | Serving size: 2 cups

This colorful soup tastes as good as it looks, and it smells great while it's cooking. The sweet potatoes and sun-dried tomatoes add an earthy sweetness and toothsome texture to this fast, easy, and delicious soup.

2 tablespoons extra-virgin olive oil

1 onion, chopped

2 carrots, peeled and chopped

1 fennel bulb, chopped

4 garlic cloves, minced

6 cups low-sodium vegetable broth

1 bunch kale, stemmed and chopped

1 (15-ounce) can white beans, drained and rinsed

½ (8-ounce) jar sun-dried tomatoes, drained and chopped

2 sweet potatoes, peeled and cut into ½-inch dice

1 tablespoon dried Italian seasoning

½ teaspoon sea salt

1. In a large pot, heat the olive oil over medium-high heat until it shimmers.
2. Add the onion, carrots, and fennel. Cook, stirring occasionally, until the vegetables are soft, about 5 minutes.
3. Add the garlic and cook, stirring constantly, for 30 seconds.
4. Add the broth, kale, white beans, tomatoes, sweet potatoes, Italian seasoning, and salt. Bring to a boil.
5. Reduce the heat to medium. Cook, stirring occasionally, until the potatoes are tender, about 10 minutes. Serve.

Per Serving: Calories: 243; Total fat: 8g; Saturated fat: 1g; Cholesterol: 0mg; Carbohydrates: 38g; Fiber: 11g; Protein: 8g; Sodium: 465mg

AVGOLEMONO SOUP

ALLERGEN-FREE, GLUTEN-FREE

Serves 6 | Prep time: 10 minutes | Cook time: 10 minutes | Serving size: 1½ cups

With bright flavors of lemon and a lovely helping of chicken, avgolemono is a simple-to-make egg and lemon soup filled with bold flavors. Consider adding a cooked grain or pasta, such as brown rice, whole-wheat orzo, or farro, to increase texture and nutritional value.

2 tablespoons extra-virgin olive oil

1 onion, minced

2 carrots, peeled and minced

2 celery stalks, minced

3 garlic cloves, minced

6 cups low-sodium chicken broth

½ teaspoon sea salt

¼ teaspoon freshly ground black pepper

2 cups shredded cooked boneless, skinless chicken breast

3 eggs, beaten

Juice of 1 lemon

1. In a large pot, heat the olive oil over medium-high heat until it shimmers.

2. Add the onion, carrots, and celery. Cook, stirring occasionally, until the vegetables are soft, about 3 minutes.

3. Add the garlic and cook, stirring constantly, for 30 seconds.

4. Add the broth, salt, and pepper. Bring to a simmer. Add the chicken and bring back to a simmer. Cook until the chicken is heated through, 2 to 3 minutes.

5. In a small bowl, use a fork to whisk together the eggs and lemon juice. While whisking, add 2 tablespoons of the hot soup.

6. Remove the pot from the heat. Pour the egg mixture in a thin stream into the soup, stirring constantly as you do. Serve.

Variation tip: You can replace the chicken with Moroccan-Spiced Turkey Meatballs (page 38) for a flavorful alternative.

Per Serving: Calories: 190; Total fat: 9g; Saturated fat: 2g; Cholesterol: 133mg; Carbohydrates: 6g; Fiber: 1g; Protein: 20g; Sodium: 360mg

TUSCAN-STYLE CHICKEN AND VEGETABLE SOUP

ALLERGEN-FREE, GLUTEN-FREE

Serves 6 | Prep time: 10 minutes | Cook time: 20 minutes | Serving size: 1½ cups

A hint of orange adds tremendous fragrance and flavor to this white bean and chicken soup. To save time, use a precooked rotisserie chicken. Or plan ahead by cooking chicken breasts, shredding them, and freezing them in 1-cup portions in zip-top bags for up to six months.

2 tablespoons extra-virgin olive oil

1 onion, chopped

2 carrots, peeled and chopped

1 fennel bulb, chopped

4 garlic cloves, minced

6 cups low-sodium chicken broth

1 tablespoon dried Italian seasoning

1 (15-ounce) can white beans, drained and rinsed

10 baby red potatoes, quartered

1 bunch kale, stemmed and chopped

Zest of ½ orange and juice of 1 orange

½ teaspoon sea salt

¼ teaspoon freshly ground black pepper

2 cups shredded cooked boneless, skinless chicken breast

¼ cup chopped Italian parsley

1. In a large pot, heat the olive oil over medium-high heat until it shimmers.

2. Add the onion, carrots, and fennel. Cook, stirring occasionally, until the vegetables are soft, about 5 minutes.

3. Add the garlic and cook, stirring constantly, for 30 seconds.

4. Add the broth, Italian seasoning, white beans, red potatoes, kale, orange juice and zest, salt, and pepper. Bring to a boil. Reduce the heat to medium and simmer, stirring occasionally, until the potatoes are tender, about 10 minutes.

5. Add the chicken and cook until it is warmed through, 1 to 2 minutes. Garnish with the parsley before serving.

Per Serving: Calories: 306; Total fat: 7g; Saturated fat: 1g; Cholesterol: 40mg; Carbohydrates: 38g; Fiber: 9g; Protein: 25g; Sodium: 560mg

CREAM OF ASPARAGUS SOUP

GLUTEN-FREE, VEGETARIAN

Serves 4 | Prep time: 10 minutes | Cook time: 20 minutes | Serving size: 2 cups

Here's your answer for using up fresh asparagus when in season. Scented with lemon and dill and thickened with Greek yogurt, asparagus is all dressed up in this this creamy, tangy vegetarian soup. Asparagus also has excellent anti-inflammatory and antioxidant properties.

2 tablespoons extra-virgin olive oil, plus a drizzle for garnish

1 onion, minced

6 cups low-sodium vegetable broth

2 bunches asparagus, trimmed and cut into 1-inch pieces

½ teaspoon sea salt

¼ teaspoon freshly ground black pepper

¼ cup chopped fresh dill

Zest and juice of 1 lemon

1 cup nonfat plain Greek yogurt

1. In a large pot, heat the olive oil over medium-high heat until it shimmers.
2. Add the onion and cook, stirring occasionally, until soft, about 3 minutes.
3. Add the broth, asparagus, salt, and pepper. Bring to a boil. Reduce the heat to medium and simmer, stirring occasionally, until the asparagus is tender, about 15 minutes.
4. Remove from the heat. Transfer the soup to a blender or food processor (or use an immersion blender). Add the dill, lemon zest and juice, and Greek yogurt. Blend until smooth.
5. Garnish with a drizzle of olive oil before serving.

Nutrition boost: This soup is already pretty heart-healthy, but you can add some texture and beneficial fats by garnishing with ½ cup of chopped almonds or walnuts.

Per Serving: Calories: 181; Total fat: 8g; Saturated fat: 1g; Cholesterol: 0mg; Carbohydrates: 21g; Fiber: 7g; Protein: 11g; Sodium: 529mg

ORANGE FENNEL LENTIL SOUP

ALLERGEN-FREE, GLUTEN-FREE, VEGAN

Serves 4 | Prep time: 10 minutes | Cook time: 15 minutes | Serving size: 2 cups

When you want something hearty, satisfying, aromatic, and fast, this is the soup for you! Canned lentils cook quickly and stick to your ribs, and in this flavorful, orange-scented broth, they take on delicious flavors.

2 tablespoons extra-virgin olive oil

1 onion, chopped

2 fennel bulbs, chopped, plus 2 tablespoons chopped fennel fronds

3 garlic cloves, minced

4 cups low-sodium vegetable broth

2 (15-ounce) cans lentils, drained

Zest and juice of 1 orange, divided

¼ teaspoon red pepper flakes (optional)

½ teaspoon sea salt

¼ teaspoon freshly ground black pepper

1. In a large pot, heat the olive oil over medium-high heat until it shimmers.
2. Add the onion and fennel bulbs and cook, stirring occasionally, until the vegetables are soft, about 5 minutes.
3. Add the garlic and cook, stirring constantly, for 30 seconds.
4. Add the broth, lentils, orange zest, red pepper flakes (if using), salt, and black pepper. Bring to a boil. Cook, stirring, for 5 minutes.
5. Remove from the heat and stir in the orange juice and fennel fronds before serving.

Nutrition boost: Because raw garlic has cardioprotective benefits, you can add delicious flavors and increase your heart health by garnishing this dish with gremolata. To make it, mix 2 minced garlic cloves, the zest of half an orange, and ½ cup of chopped fresh parsley.

Per Serving: Calories: 343; Total fat: 7g; Saturated fat: 1g; Cholesterol: 0mg; Carbohydrates: 52g; Fiber: 19g; Protein: 18g; Sodium: 914mg

TURKEY GYRO MEATBALL SOUP

ALLERGEN-FREE, GLUTEN-FREE

Serves 4 | Prep time: 15 minutes | Cook time: 25 minutes | Serving size: 2 cups

If you love the classic Greek sandwiches called gyros, you'll be salivating over this soup. The turkey meatballs are filled with Greek flavors and spices, making for a satisfying and fragrant hot bowl of soup.

1 pound ground turkey breast

1 onion, grated and the water squeezed out (see Ingredient tip)

¼ cup chopped fresh rosemary

¼ cup chopped fresh parsley

¼ cup chopped fresh oregano

6 garlic cloves, minced, divided

2 tablespoons extra-virgin olive oil

1 red onion, chopped

2 carrots, peeled and chopped

6 cups low-sodium chicken broth

1. In a large bowl, combine the turkey, onion, rosemary, parsley, oregano, and 4 minced garlic cloves. Form into 1-inch meatballs.

2. In a large pot, heat the olive oil over medium-high heat until it shimmers.

3. Add the onion and carrots and cook, stirring occasionally, until the vegetables are soft, about 5 minutes.

4. Add the remaining 2 minced garlic cloves and cook, stirring constantly, for 30 seconds.

5. Add the broth. Bring to a boil.

6. Add the meatballs. Boil until the meatballs are cooked, about 15 minutes. Serve.

Ingredient tip: To squeeze all the water out of the onion, wrap the grated onion in a tea towel and wring until all the water comes out. If you have a food processor, you can use it to combine the squeezed-out onions, garlic, herbs, and ground turkey to mix it well.

Per Serving: Calories: 247; Total fat: 9g; Saturated fat: 2g; Cholesterol: 55mg; Carbohydrates: 11g; Fiber: 2g; Protein: 31g; Sodium: 495mg

GREEK TURKEY, VEGGIE, AND ORZO SOUP

ALLERGEN-FREE

Serves 4 | Prep time: 15 minutes | Cook time: 20 minutes | Serving size: 2 cups

Lemon and garlic scent this delicious ground turkey soup. It's an easy soup to customize—so if you have veggies you want to add, go for it! They will only enhance this delicious and easy-to-make soup.

2 tablespoons extra-virgin olive oil

1 pound ground turkey breast

1 onion, chopped

2 carrots, peeled and chopped

3 garlic cloves, minced

4 cups low-sodium chicken broth

1 (15-ounce) can chickpeas, drained and rinsed

1 cup whole-wheat orzo

1 teaspoon dried oregano

Zest and juice of 1 lemon, divided

½ teaspoon sea salt

4 cups baby spinach

1. In a large pot, heat the olive oil over medium-high heat until it shimmers.
2. Add the turkey and cook, crumbling, until browned, about 5 minutes. Using a slotted spoon, remove the turkey and set aside.
3. Add the onion and carrots to the rendered fat in the pot and cook, stirring occasionally, until the vegetables are soft, about 5 minutes.
4. Add the garlic and cook, stirring constantly, for 30 seconds.
5. Add the broth, chickpeas, orzo, oregano, lemon zest, and salt. Bring to a boil. Reduce the heat to medium and simmer, stirring occasionally, until the orzo is tender, about 6 minutes.
6. Add the spinach and return the turkey to the pot. Cook, stirring, for 2 minutes more.
7. Remove from the heat and stir in the lemon juice before serving.

Substitution tip: To make this gluten-free, substitute gluten-free orzo or use 2 cups of cooked brown rice instead.

Per Serving: Calories: 487; Total fat: 10g; Saturated fat: 2g; Cholesterol: 55mg; Carbohydrates: 58g; Fiber: 8g; Protein: 40g; Sodium: 610mg

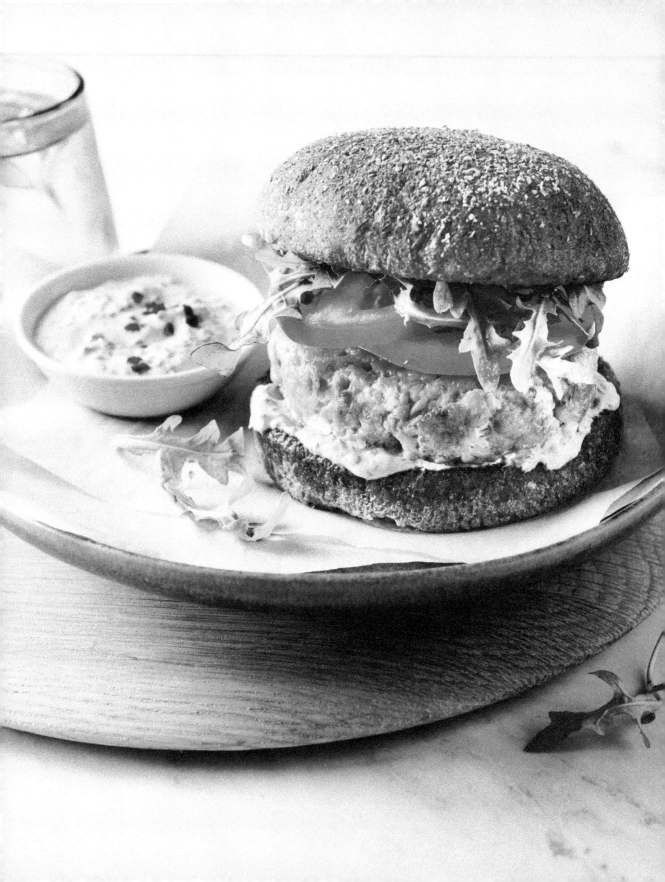

— CHAPTER 5 —

SANDWICHES AND SPREADS

< Moroccan-Spiced Turkey Burgers with Chermoula Yogurt, page 79

WHITE BEAN DIP

ALLERGEN-FREE, GLUTEN-FREE, VEGAN

Serves 6 | Prep time: 5 minutes | Serving size: ¼ cup

Fiber- and magnesium-rich white beans make an oh-so-flavorful creamy dip with garlic, rosemary, and orange flavors. This dip is perfect on a veggie sandwich or as a spread for your favorite turkey burger, or you can use it as a delicious and nutritious dip for pita chips or veggies.

2 (14-ounce) cans white beans, drained and rinsed

2 garlic cloves, minced

2 tablespoons chopped fresh rosemary

4 tablespoons extra-virgin olive oil, divided

Juice of 1 orange

½ teaspoon sea salt

1. In a blender or food processor, combine the beans, garlic, rosemary, 3 tablespoons of olive oil, orange juice, and salt.
2. Blend until smooth.
3. Drizzle the remaining 1 tablespoon of olive oil as a garnish before serving.

Per Serving: Calories: 203; Total fat: 9g; Saturated fat: 1g; Cholesterol: 0mg; Carbohydrates: 25g; Fiber: 8g; Protein: 8g; Sodium: 352mg

TZATZIKI

GLUTEN-FREE, VEGETARIAN

Serves 4 | Prep time: 10 minutes, plus 1 hour to chill | Serving size: ¼ cup

A tangy, yogurt-based sauce, tzatziki is a refreshing dip or spread that's equally delicious on sandwiches or gyros or as a dip for veggies or pita chips. With fragrant herbs and refreshing cucumber, this creamy concoction is bound to become a new family favorite.

1 medium cucumber, grated

2½ cups nonfat plain Greek yogurt

1 garlic clove, minced

2 tablespoons chopped fresh dill

Juice of ½ lemon

3 tablespoons extra-virgin olive oil

½ teaspoon sea salt

1. Wrap the grated cucumber in a tea towel and wring out the excess water.
2. In a medium bowl, combine the cucumber, yogurt, garlic, dill, lemon juice, olive oil, and salt.
3. Stir to combine. Refrigerate for 1 hour before serving.

Substitution tip: Make this vegan and/or dairy-free by using 1½ cups of plain nondairy yogurt and adding ½ cup of olive oil mayonnaise or vegan mayonnaise.

Per Serving: Calories: 168; Total fat: 11g; Saturated fat: 2g; Cholesterol: 0mg; Carbohydrates: 7; Fiber: 1g; Protein: 12g; Sodium: 338mg

TAPENADE

ALLERGEN-FREE, GLUTEN-FREE, VEGAN

Serves 6 | Prep time: 10 minutes, plus 2 hours to chill | Serving size: ¼ cup

Tapenade—a delicious dip, sandwich spread, or topping for fish and poultry—is a popular Mediterranean diet staple. Table olives, especially Kalamata olives, are rich sources of antioxidant polyphenols benefiting heart health. If you don't have a food processor, you can finely chop all the ingredients by hand.

1 cup Kalamata olives, pitted

½ cup Spanish olives, pitted

2 garlic cloves

¼ teaspoon red pepper flakes

¼ cup fresh Italian parsley

¼ cup fresh rosemary

2 tablespoons extra-virgin olive oil

½ teaspoon sea salt

1. In a food processor, combine the Kalamata olives, Spanish olives, garlic, red pepper flakes, parsley, rosemary, olive oil, and salt.
2. Pulse for 20 one-second pulses, or until the pieces of olives and herbs are very small.
3. Refrigerate for 2 hours before serving.

Nutritional boost: Boost heart-healthy fats by replacing half of the Kalamata olives with ½ cup of finely chopped almonds.

Per Serving: Calories: 104; Total fat: 10g; Saturated fat: 1g; Cholesterol: 0mg; Carbohydrates: 3g; Fiber: <1g; Protein: <1g; Sodium: 594mg

HUMMUS, KALE, AND QUICK-PICKLED ONION PITAS

ALLERGEN-FREE, GLUTEN-FREE, VEGAN

Serves 4 | Prep time: 1 hour 10 minutes | Serving size: 2 pita halves

A red onion quick pickle adds a delicious acidic bite to this sandwich that pairs well with the creamy, spicy hummus. You can use homemade hummus or choose your favorite store-bought brand.

½ cup red wine vinegar

1 teaspoon sea salt

1 (1-gram) packet stevia

½ red onion, thinly sliced

4 whole-wheat pitas, halved

1 cup Easy Hummus (page 32) or store-bought hummus

2 cups chopped kale

1 cup cherry tomatoes, halved

½ (12-ounce) jar roasted red peppers, drained and chopped

1. In a small bowl, combine the red wine vinegar, salt, and stevia. Submerge the onion in the pickling liquid. Cover and allow to sit at room temperature for 1 hour, then drain.

2. Inside each pita half, spread 2 tablespoons of hummus.

3. Divide the kale, red onion, tomatoes, and roasted red peppers between the pita halves. Serve.

Nutritional boost: Add 2 tablespoons of pepitas to the hummus to add heart-healthy nutrients and fats.

Per Serving: Calories: 322; Total fat: 15g; Saturated fat: 2g; Cholesterol: 0mg; Carbohydrates: 44g; Fiber: 9g; Protein: 12g; Sodium: 991mg

TURKEY MUFFULETTA

Serves 6 | Prep time: 15 minutes, plus up to 1 day to rest | Serving size: ⅙ sandwich

A muffuletta is a hearty, savory sandwich that's made for the whole family. You'll use a whole focaccia and cut it into wedges to serve a crowd. Letting it rest for an hour in the fridge allows the bread to soak up the juices from the sandwich, but you can skip this step if you want to eat it right away.

1 loaf whole-wheat focaccia, split

1 recipe Tapenade (page 68)

1 (12-ounce) jar roasted red peppers, drained and chopped

½ cup jarred pepperoncini or banana peppers, drained and chopped

¼ cup chopped fresh basil

4 ounces thinly sliced deli turkey

4 ounces thinly sliced turkey ham

4 ounces sliced Havarti cheese (or your cheese of choice)

1. Scoop out some of the bread from the cut sides of the focaccia to accommodate the sandwich fillings.

2. On the bottom half, spread the tapenade in an even layer.

3. Spread the roasted red peppers and pepperoncini in even layers over the tapenade.

4. Sprinkle with the basil.

5. Add a layer of turkey and a layer of turkey ham.

6. Top with a layer of Havarti and the other half of the focaccia.

7. Press the sandwich between two plates or wrap it in plastic and refrigerate for up to one day.

8. Cut into wedges to serve.

Substitution tip: You can make this vegan by omitting the turkey and turkey ham. Instead, add 8 ounces of thinly sliced seitan, and replace the cheese with vegan cheese slices. You can add more flavor by sprinkling with 1 cup of sun-dried tomatoes.

Per Serving: Calories: 405; Total fat: 18g; Saturated fat: 3g; Cholesterol: 28mg; Carbohydrates: 44g; Fiber: 3g; Protein: 20g; Sodium: 1,462mg

TUNA AND ROASTED RED PEPPER SANDWICHES

Serves 2 | Prep time: 10 minutes | Serving size: 1 sandwich

Omega-3-rich albacore tuna tastes even better when it's combined with Mediterranean flavors such as roasted red peppers, capers, and lemon. These sandwiches are fast and easy to make, and the tuna salad will keep well in the fridge for about three days.

1 (5-ounce) can water-packed albacore tuna, drained

½ (12-ounce) jar roasted red peppers, drained and chopped

2 tablespoons capers, drained and rinsed

½ fennel bulb, finely chopped

½ cup chopped black olives

¼ cup nonfat plain Greek yogurt

1 tablespoon freshly squeezed lemon juice

½ teaspoon grated lemon zest

2 tablespoons chopped fresh dill

¼ teaspoon sea salt

4 slices whole-wheat bread

1. In a small bowl, combine the tuna, roasted red peppers, capers, fennel, and olives.
2. In another bowl, mix together the yogurt, lemon juice, lemon zest, dill, and salt.
3. Mix the dressing with the tuna salad.
4. Spread on 2 slices of bread and top with the other 2 slices. Serve.

Variation tip: This is also very good with canned salmon, which is also a heart-healthy fish.

Per Serving: Calories: 406; Total fat: 12g; Saturated fat: 0g; Cholesterol: 25mg; Carbohydrates: 57g; Fiber: 14g; Protein: 30g; Sodium: 1,507mg

EGG SALAD SANDWICHES WITH PEPPERONCINI

VEGETARIAN

Serves 2 | Prep time: 10 minutes | Serving size: 1 sandwich

Spicy pepperoncini add a bit of gentle heat, some acidity, and lots of texture to these egg salad sandwiches. If you have a pickled pepper you like better, it's a perfectly acceptable substitute, so feel free to play a little with the seasonings and veggies to make them suit your palate.

5 hard-boiled eggs, finely chopped (see Ingredient tip on page 24)

½ cup jarred pepperoncini, drained and finely chopped

½ cup sun-dried tomatoes, finely chopped

¼ cup chopped fresh basil

1 tablespoon nonfat plain Greek yogurt

3 tablespoons Easy Hummus (page 32) or store-bought hummus

¼ teaspoon sea salt

4 slices whole-grain bread, toasted

1. In a medium bowl, combine the eggs, pepperoncini, tomatoes, and basil.
2. In another bowl, whisk together the yogurt, hummus, and salt.
3. Mix the dressing with the salad.
4. Spread on 2 slices of the toasted bread and top with the other 2 slices. Serve.

Nutritional boost: **You can make this heart-healthier by using 2 whole hard-boiled eggs along with just the whites of 4 more hard-boiled eggs. Alternatively, you can replace 2 eggs with ¼ cup of chopped extra-firm tofu.**

Per Serving: Calories: 493; Total fat: 21g; Saturated fat: 5g; Cholesterol: 465mg; Carbohydrates: 55g; Fiber: 13g; Protein: 30g; Sodium: 1,337mg

OPEN-FACED SHRIMP, FENNEL, AND CHEESE SANDWICHES

Serves 2 | Prep time: 10 minutes | Cook time: 5 minutes | Serving size: 1 sandwich

Shrimp and fennel make a beautiful flavor combination. Fennel adds a fresh, light anise flavor that blends well with sweet shrimp while adding texture and crunch. The mild cheese melts over the top, creating a warm, delicious sandwich.

6 ounces cooked baby shrimp

½ bulb fennel, finely chopped, plus 2 tablespoons finely chopped fennel fronds

½ (12-ounce) jar roasted red peppers, drained and chopped

¼ cup nonfat, plain Greek yogurt

¼ teaspoon sea salt

2 slices whole-wheat bread, toasted

2 slices Swiss cheese

1. Preheat the oven's broiler on high.
2. In a medium bowl, combine the shrimp, fennel bulb and fronds, roasted red peppers, yogurt, and salt. Mix well.
3. Place the toasted bread side by side on a baking sheet. Spoon the shrimp mixture onto the bread and top with the cheese.
4. Broil until the cheese is melted and starts to brown, about 4 minutes. Let cool slightly before serving.

Substitution tip: If you're allergic to shellfish but not fish, you can make this sandwich with 1 (5-ounce) can of drained albacore tuna or 1 (5-ounce) can of drained salmon.

Per Serving: Calories: 311; Total fat: 8g; Saturated fat: 3g; Cholesterol: 185mg; Carbohydrates: 32g; Fiber: 8g; Protein: 32g; Sodium: 724mg

SALMON AND TAPENADE PITAS

Serves 2 | Prep time: 10 minutes | Serving size: 1 pita

Mixing heart-healthy salmon with tapenade makes a delicious, flavorful, moist filling for pitas. Add some veggies for crunch and a little lemon and Greek yogurt for creaminess and flavor, and you've got a satisfying pita sandwich.

1 (5-ounce) can salmon, drained and rinsed

1 recipe Tapenade (page 68)

1 celery stalk, minced

½ red bell pepper, seeded and finely chopped

3 scallions, thinly sliced

2 tablespoons nonfat plain Greek yogurt

¼ teaspoon grated lemon zest, plus 1 teaspoon freshly squeezed lemon juice

¼ teaspoon sea salt

2 whole-wheat pitas, halved

1. In a small bowl, combine the salmon, tapenade, celery, bell pepper, scallions, yogurt, lemon zest, and juice, and salt. Mix well.
2. Spoon into the pita halves. Serve.

Substitution tip: If you are allergic to fish but not shellfish, you can use 1½ cups of baby shrimp in place of the salmon. If you're allergic to both, you can use 1½ cups of chopped cooked boneless, skinless chicken breast.

Per Serving: Calories: 536; Total fat: 33g; Saturated fat: 3g; Cholesterol: 20mg; Carbohydrates: 41g; Fiber: 6g; Protein: 21g; Sodium: 2,466mg

TURKEY HAM, ROASTED RED PEPPER, AND CHEESE PANINI

Serves 1 | Prep time: 10 minutes | Cook time: 10 minutes | Serving size: 1 sandwich

Panini are delicious with their melted cheese and savory fillings. You don't need a special pan to make them. Instead, you can place something heavy (and heatproof) on the panini as it cooks to press the sandwich.

2 slices whole-wheat bread

3 tablespoons extra-virgin olive oil

3 ounces deli-sliced turkey ham

⅓ (12-ounce) jar roasted red peppers

4 basil leaves, chopped

¼ cup grated Swiss cheese

1. Heat a panini press, grill pan, or skillet over medium-high heat.
2. Brush both sides of the bread with the olive oil.
3. Place the turkey ham and roasted red peppers on 1 slice of bread. Sprinkle with the basil and top with the cheese and the other slice of bread.
4. Place into your hot pan. Press while cooking. Cook on both sides until browned, about 4 minutes per side. Let cool slightly before serving.

Ingredient tip: To press the panini, you can use a countertop electric grill. If you're using a skillet on the stovetop, use a large skillet. Place a heatproof plate on top of the sandwich and weight it with something heavy, such as a large can of beans or tomatoes.

Per Serving: Calories: 768; Total fat: 55g; Saturated fat: 11g; Cholesterol: 64mg; Carbohydrates: 47g; Fiber: 10g; Protein: 31g; Sodium: 1,325mg

CHICKEN AND GREEK SALAD SANDWICH WRAPS WITH TZATZIKI

Serves 4 | Prep time: 10 minutes | Serving size: 1 wrap

This recipe is especially good if you have leftover salad and cooked chicken breast. You can save time by purchasing a precooked rotisserie chicken breast at the grocery store. Just remove the skin and bones.

1 cup Tzatziki (page 67)

4 large whole-wheat tortillas or sandwich wraps

2 cups chopped cooked boneless, skinless chicken breast

4 cups Easy Greek Salad (page 46)

1. Spread ¼ cup of tzatziki on each tortilla.
2. Top each with ½ cup of chicken and 1 cup of salad.
3. Wrap and serve.

Per Serving: Calories: 600; Total fat: 34g; Saturated fat: 7g; Cholesterol: 77mg; Carbohydrates: 40g; Fiber: 10g; Protein: 39g; Sodium: 1,164mg

TURKEY, AVOCADO, AND FETA SANDWICH WRAPS

Serves 4 | Prep time: 10 minutes | Serving size: 1 wrap

Protein-rich turkey breast paired with avocado's heart-healthy monounsaturated fat is an impeccable match. These mouthwatering wraps are a tasty and fun alternative to traditional sandwiches, ideal for a quick work or school lunch.

1 avocado, peeled, pitted, and mashed

1 teaspoon freshly squeezed lemon juice

¼ cup nonfat plain Greek yogurt

½ teaspoon sea salt

1 tablespoon chopped fresh dill

2 cups chopped cooked turkey breast

4 whole-wheat tortillas or sandwich wraps

1 cup cherry tomatoes, halved

½ cup crumbled feta cheese

1. In a small bowl, mash together the avocado, lemon juice, yogurt, salt, and dill. Fold in the turkey breast.
2. Spread the mixture on the sandwich wraps.
3. Sprinkle with the tomatoes and feta cheese.
4. Wrap and serve.

Ingredient tip: To easily peel and pit an avocado, cut the avocado lengthwise around the pit. Use a knife to remove the pit. Then, use a large spoon to scoop out the avocado flesh.

Per Serving: Calories: 368; Total fat: 16g; Saturated fat: 5g; Cholesterol: 67mg; Carbohydrates: 35g; Fiber: 6g; Protein: 27g; Sodium: 1,852mg

GREEK-STYLE CHICKEN SALAD SANDWICHES

Serves 4 | Prep time: 10 minutes | Serving size: 2 pita halves

With savory and spicy Greek flavors, these aren't your average chicken salad sandwiches. You can make the chicken salad ahead of time and then spread it on your favorite bread, wrap it, or put it in a pita for an easy and quick lunch.

2 cups chopped cooked boneless, skinless chicken breast

1 small cucumber, diced

½ red onion, finely chopped

½ cup chopped black olives

½ cup crumbled feta cheese

1 cup grape tomatoes, halved

¼ cup chopped fresh oregano

¼ cup nonfat plain Greek yogurt

Juice of ½ lemon

1 garlic clove, minced

¼ teaspoon sea salt

4 whole-wheat pitas, halved

1. In a large bowl, combine the chicken, cucumber, onion, olives, cheese, tomatoes, and oregano.
2. In a small bowl, whisk together the Greek yogurt, lemon juice, garlic, and sea salt.
3. Mix the dressing with the salad and spoon into the pita halves. Serve.

Substitution tip: To make these gluten-free, you can roll the chicken salad in large pieces of butter lettuce or simply eat it as a salad.

Per Serving: Calories: 389; Total fat: 10g; Saturated fat: 4g; Cholesterol: 76mg; Carbohydrates: 43g; Fiber: 4g; Protein: 33g; Sodium: 833mg

MOROCCAN-SPICED TURKEY BURGERS WITH CHERMOULA YOGURT

Serves 4 | Prep time: 10 minutes | Cook time: 15 minutes | Serving size: 1 burger

If your favorite sandwich is a burger, then you'll love these delicious and fragrant burgers topped with ultra-flavorful chermoula yogurt. While this recipe calls for buns, you can up your Mediterranean cuisine cred by serving them in toasty pitas.

1 pound ground turkey breast

1¼ teaspoons ground cumin, divided

½ teaspoon ground cinnamon

4 garlic cloves, minced, divided

¾ teaspoon sea salt, divided

Nonstick cooking spray

½ cup nonfat plain Greek yogurt

½ cup chopped fresh cilantro

½ cup chopped fresh mint

¼ teaspoon ground coriander

¼ teaspoon grated lemon zest

¼ teaspoon paprika

¼ teaspoon red pepper flakes

4 whole-wheat hamburger buns, split and toasted

1. In a large bowl, combine the turkey breast, 1 teaspoon of cumin, cinnamon, 3 minced garlic cloves, and ½ teaspoon of salt. Form into four patties.

2. Spray a large nonstick pan with cooking spray and heat over medium-high heat. Place the burgers in the pan and cook until cooked through, 5 to 7 minutes per side.

3. While the burgers cook, in a small bowl, combine the Greek yogurt, remaining ¼ teaspoon of cumin, remaining 1 minced garlic clove, remaining ¼ teaspoon of salt, cilantro, mint, coriander, lemon zest, paprika, and red pepper flakes. Mix well.

4. Spread the sauce on the cut sides of the buns and assemble the burgers. Serve.

Ingredient tip: Add more flavor and texture to these burgers by topping with arugula and sliced tomatoes.

Per Serving: Calories: 280; Total fat: 4g; Saturated fat: 1g; Cholesterol: 55mg; Carbohydrates: 28g; Fiber: 5g; Protein: 36g; Sodium: 718mg

MEATBALL PITAS WITH CREAMY PESTO

Serves 4 | Prep time: 20 minutes | Cook time: 30 minutes | Serving size: 2 pita halves

Pesto is such a fresh, flavorful addition to any food, and in these pitas, it adds bright flavors to savory meatballs. The meatballs also freeze well, so feel free to make a big batch and freeze them in single servings in freezer bags.

½ cup skim milk

½ cup whole-wheat bread crumbs

1 pound bulk Italian turkey sausage

4 garlic cloves, minced, divided

1 tablespoon dried Italian seasoning

1 egg, beaten

½ cup basil leaves

¼ cup pine nuts

¼ cup grated Parmesan cheese

¼ cup extra-virgin olive oil

¼ cup nonfat plain Greek yogurt

4 whole-wheat pitas, halved

1. Preheat the oven to 400°F. Line a rimmed baking sheet with parchment paper and set aside.
2. In a large bowl, combine the milk and bread crumbs. Allow to sit for 10 minutes.
3. Stir the milk and bread crumbs. Add the sausage, 2 minced garlic cloves, Italian seasoning, and egg. Mix well.
4. Roll the mixture into 1-inch balls. Place the meatballs on the prepared baking sheet.
5. Bake until the internal temperature reaches 165°F, 20 to 30 minutes.
6. While the meatballs cook, in a blender or food processor, combine the basil, pine nuts, Parmesan cheese, olive oil, and the remaining 2 minced garlic cloves. Process for 20 one-second pulses.
7. Put the yogurt into a small bowl and fold the pesto into the yogurt.
8. To make the sandwiches, divide the meatballs between the pita halves and spoon the yogurt-pesto sauce over the top. Serve.

Nutritional boost: Add heart-healthy lycopene by chopping 1 large tomato and adding it to the pitas.

Per Serving: Calories: 671; Total fat: 37g; Saturated fat: 8g; Cholesterol: 122mg; Carbohydrates: 54g; Fiber: 3g; Protein: 31g; Sodium: 1,587mg

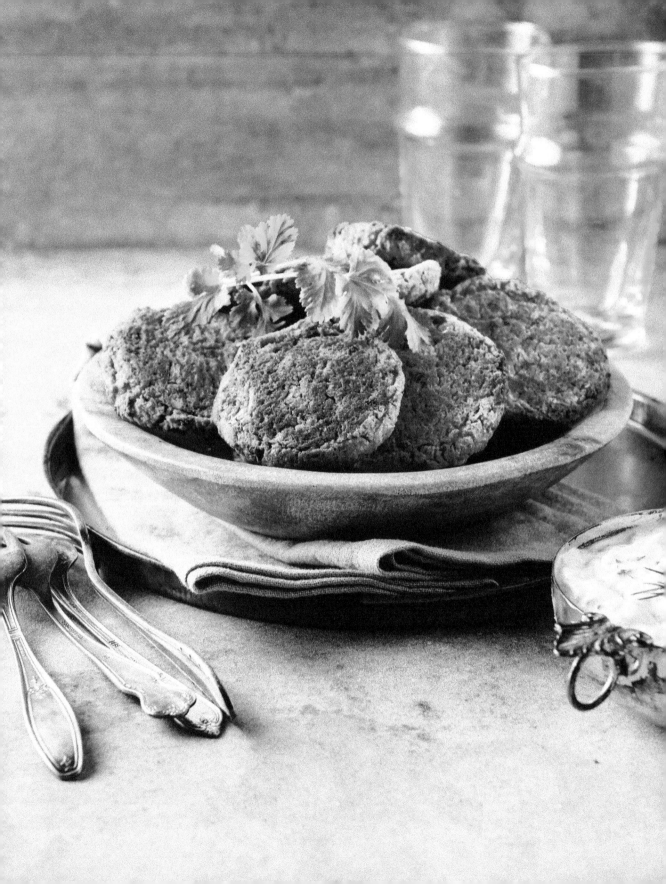

CHAPTER 6

VEGETARIAN AND VEGAN ENTRÉES

< Falafel with Tzatziki, page 84

FALAFEL WITH TZATZIKI

VEGETARIAN

Serves 6 | **Prep time: 10 minutes** | **Cook time: 25 minutes** | **Serving size: 2 falafel and ¼ cup tzatziki**

These falafel patties are flavorful and delicious, and the creamy, cool tzatziki adds the perfect counterpoint to the crunchy spice of the falafel. You can use falafel in a pita to make a sandwich, serve it on a bed of greens with chopped tomato, or enjoy it as a main dish all by itself.

4 tablespoons extra-virgin olive oil, divided, plus more for greasing

2 (15-ounce) cans chickpeas, drained and rinsed

½ onion, finely chopped

5 garlic cloves, minced

½ cup fresh cilantro

1½ teaspoons ground cumin

1½ teaspoon ground coriander

Juice of ½ lemon

½ teaspoon sea salt

¼ teaspoon freshly ground black pepper

2 tablespoons whole-wheat flour

1 recipe Tzatziki (page 67)

1. Preheat the oven to 375°F. Line a baking sheet with parchment paper and brush the parchment with olive oil. Set aside.

2. In a blender or food processor, combine 2 tablespoons of olive oil, the chickpeas, onion, garlic, cilantro, cumin, coriander, lemon juice, salt, pepper, and flour. Process for 20 one-second pulses until well chopped and combined.

3. Roll the mixture into 12 balls and then flatten them into patties. Place the patties on the prepared baking sheet and brush the tops with the remaining 2 tablespoons of olive oil.

4. Bake for about 25 minutes, flipping the falafel halfway through, until the falafel are crisp and brown.

5. Serve hot, topped with the tzatziki.

Substitution tip: To make this dish gluten-free, replace the wheat flour with almond flour.

Per Serving: Calories: 351; Total fat: 18g; Saturated fat: 3g; Cholesterol: 0mg; Carbohydrates: 35g; Fiber: 8g; Protein: 16g; Sodium: 587mg

EGGPLANT PARMESAN STACKS

VEGETARIAN

Serves 4 | Prep time: 10 minutes | Cook time: 15 minutes | Serving size: 1 stack and ¼ cup sauce

Cutting the eggplant into very thin slices (about ¼ inch thick) results in a crisper texture that adds a toothsome bite to the sweet tomato sauce and savory cheese.

1½ cups whole-wheat bread crumbs

1 eggplant, cut into ¼-inch-thick slices

2 eggs, beaten

2 tablespoons extra-virgin olive oil

½ onion, finely chopped

4 garlic cloves, minced

1 (28-ounce) can crushed tomatoes

1 tablespoon dried Italian seasoning

½ teaspoon sea salt

¼ teaspoon red pepper flakes

4 ounces grated Parmesan cheese

¼ cup chopped fresh basil

1. Preheat the oven to 400°F.
2. Spread the bread crumbs on a plate.
3. Dip the eggplant slices in the egg and then in the bread crumbs to coat. Place in a single layer on one or more rimmed baking sheets as needed.
4. Bake for 12 minutes, flipping halfway through.
5. While the eggplant bakes, in a large skillet, heat the olive oil over medium-high heat until it shimmers.
6. Add the onion and cook, stirring occasionally, until soft, about 3 minutes.
7. Add the garlic and cook, stirring constantly, for 30 seconds.
8. Add the tomatoes with their juices, Italian seasoning, salt, and red pepper flakes. Bring to a simmer. Reduce the heat to medium-low and cook, stirring occasionally, for 10 minutes.
9. To assemble, layer the eggplant slices and the sauce in four equal stacks, spooning any remaining sauce over the top of the stacks. Garnish with the Parmesan cheese and basil before serving.

Ingredient tip: It's best to salt the eggplant ahead of time to remove bitter fluids. To do this, place the sliced eggplant in a colander and sprinkle liberally with sea salt. Allow it to drain for 30 minutes. Rinse off the salt and pat dry.

Per Serving: Calories: 435; Total fat: 18g; Saturated fat: 7g; Cholesterol: 115mg; Carbohydrates: 47g; Fiber: 7g; Protein: 27g; Sodium: 1,184mg

STUFFED ZUCCHINI

GLUTEN-FREE, VEGAN

Serves 4 | Prep time: 10 minutes | Cook time: 40 minutes
Serving size: 2 zucchini halves and 1 cup filling

A savory vegetable and lentil ragout stuffs these boats, making them a delicious and hearty meal. The zucchini is tender while the sauce is fragrant. These freeze well and can be reheated in the microwave.

4 medium zucchini, halved lengthwise and a small amount of the flesh scooped out

2 tablespoons extra-virgin olive oil

1 red onion, chopped

1 red bell pepper, stemmed and chopped

1 fennel bulb, chopped

8 ounces shiitake mushrooms, sliced

4 garlic cloves, minced

1 (15-ounce) can crushed tomatoes

1 (15-ounce) can lentils, drained and rinsed

1 tablespoon dried Italian seasoning

½ teaspoon sea salt

¼ teaspoon red pepper flakes

1. Preheat the oven to 400°F. Line a baking sheet with parchment paper.
2. Place the zucchini halves, cut-side up, on the prepared baking sheet.
3. In a large pot, heat the olive oil over medium-high heat until it shimmers.
4. Add the onion, bell pepper, fennel, and mushrooms and cook, stirring occasionally, until the vegetables begin to brown, about 5 minutes.
5. Add the garlic and cook, stirring constantly, for 30 seconds.
6. Add the tomatoes with their juices, lentils, Italian seasoning, salt, and red pepper flakes. Bring to a simmer. Cook, stirring occasionally, for 5 minutes.
7. Spoon the mixture into the zucchini boats. Bake until the zucchini are soft, about 25 minutes. Serve.

Per Serving: Calories: 290; Total fat: 8g; Saturated fat: 1g; Cholesterol: 0mg; Carbohydrates: 46g; Fiber: 15g; Protein: 16g; Sodium: 687mg

MOROCCAN-SPICED LENTIL STEW

VEGAN
—

Serves 6 | Prep time: 10 minutes | Cook time: 20 minutes | Serving size: 1½ cups

In addition to the heart-healthy support from lentils, this stew is fragrant, warm, and savory. It makes a satisfying, stick-to-your-ribs winter meal, and it freezes very well, so you can take leftover portions with you for a healthy lunch.

2 tablespoons extra-virgin olive oil

1 onion, finely chopped

3 carrots, peeled and chopped

2 red bell peppers, seeded and roughly chopped

3 garlic cloves, minced

2 tablespoons whole-wheat flour

3 cups low-sodium vegetable broth

1 (15-ounce) can crushed tomatoes, drained

2 (15-ounce) cans lentils, drained and rinsed

1 teaspoon ground cumin

1 teaspoon ground coriander

1 teaspoon ground cinnamon

½ teaspoon sea salt

1 cup whole-wheat orzo, cooked according to package instructions

1. In a large pot, heat the olive oil over medium-high heat until it shimmers.

2. Add the onion, carrots, and bell peppers and cook, stirring occasionally, until the vegetables are tender, about 4 minutes.

3. Add the garlic and cook, stirring constantly, for 30 seconds.

4. Add the flour and cook, stirring, for 1 minute.

5. Add the broth and use the side of a spoon to scrape any browned bits from the bottom of the pan. Add the tomatoes, lentils, cumin, coriander, cinnamon, and salt. Bring to a boil and reduce the heat to medium. Cook, stirring occasionally, until the vegetables are tender, about 10 minutes.

6. Stir in the cooked orzo. Cook, stirring, for 2 minutes more. Serve.

Nutritional boost: Add heart-healthy leafy greens by adding 2 cups of chopped kale or Swiss chard in step 5. To make this gluten-free, omit the flour and replace the orzo with cooked brown rice.

Per Serving: Calories: 348; Total fat: 5g; Saturated fat: 1g; Cholesterol: 0mg; Carbohydrates: 58g; Fiber: 14g; Protein: 18g; Sodium: 654mg

MEDITERRANEAN WHITE BEAN CHILI

VEGAN

Serves 6 | Prep time: 10 minutes | Cook time: 15 minutes | Serving size: 1½ cups

Chili always makes a hearty meal, and this white bean version has delicious, warm spices. Make a double batch and freeze it in single-serving sizes for a quick reheat in the microwave when you have busy days with limited time to cook lunch or dinner.

2 tablespoons extra-virgin olive oil

1 red onion, finely chopped

1 red bell pepper, seeded and roughly chopped

4 garlic cloves, minced

3 tablespoons whole-wheat flour

6 cups low-sodium vegetable broth

2 (15-ounce) cans white beans, drained and rinsed

1 teaspoon ground cumin

1 teaspoon dried ground oregano

½ teaspoon ground allspice

½ teaspoon sea salt

¼ teaspoon freshly ground black pepper

2 tablespoons chopped fresh cilantro

1. In a large pot, heat the olive oil over medium-high heat until it shimmers.
2. Add the onion and bell pepper and cook, stirring occasionally, until the vegetables begin to brown, about 5 minutes.
3. Add the garlic and cook, stirring constantly, for 30 seconds.
4. Add the flour and cook, stirring, for 1 minute.
5. Add the broth and use the side of a spoon to scrape any browned bits from the bottom of the pan.
6. Add the beans, cumin, oregano, allspice, salt, and black pepper. Bring to a boil, stirring occasionally. Reduce the heat to medium and continue cooking for 5 minutes more, stirring occasionally.
7. Serve garnished with the cilantro.

Substitution tip: You can use any gluten-free flour in place of the regular flour to make this gluten- and allergen-free.

Per Serving: Calories: 191; Total fat: 5g; Saturated fat: 1g; Cholesterol: 0mg; Carbohydrates: 32g; Fiber: 9g; Protein: 9g; Sodium: 651mg

SWEET POTATO AND CHICKPEA STEW

VEGAN

Serves 6 | Prep time: 10 minutes | Cook time: 20 minutes | Serving size: 2 cups

Here's a combo your heart will love: potassium-rich sweet potatoes and chickpeas in a lightly spicy stew. You can also use 3 cups of cubed butternut squash in place of the sweet potatoes for a slightly different flavor profile in this tasty and hearty meal.

2 tablespoons extra-virgin olive oil

1 onion, finely chopped

2 carrots, peeled and chopped

3 garlic cloves, minced

3 tablespoons whole-wheat flour

4 cups low-sodium vegetable broth

2 sweet potatoes, peeled and cut into ½-inch cubes

2 (15-ounce) cans chickpeas, drained and rinsed

1 (15-ounce) can chopped tomatoes, drained

½ teaspoon ground cinnamon

1 teaspoon ground cumin

½ teaspoon sea salt

1. In a large pot, heat the olive oil over medium-high heat until it shimmers.
2. Add the onion and carrots and cook, stirring occasionally, until the vegetables begin to brown, about 5 minutes.
3. Add the garlic and cook, stirring constantly, for 30 seconds.
4. Add the flour and cook, stirring, for 1 minute.
5. Add the broth and use the side of a spoon to scrape any browned bits from the bottom of the pan.
6. Add the sweet potatoes, chickpeas, tomatoes, cinnamon, cumin, and salt. Bring to a boil. Reduce the heat to medium and simmer, stirring occasionally, until the potatoes are soft, about 10 minutes. Serve.

Nutritional boost: Add heart-healthy fiber by serving this with ¼ cup of brown rice, barley, or farro.

Per Serving: Calories: 277; Total fat: 6g; Saturated fat: 1g; Cholesterol: 0mg; Carbohydrates: 48g; Fiber: 11g; Protein: 9g; Sodium: 548mg

PASTA ROMESCO

VEGAN

Serves 4 | Prep time: 10 minutes | Serving size: 1 cup pasta and ¼ cup sauce

Romesco sauce is a classic tomato-based sauce. Bold and zippy, this sauce is delicious on pasta but also yummy when used as a spread for sandwiches, on eggs for breakfast, or even as a dip for fresh veggies.

1 (12-ounce) jar roasted red peppers, drained

¼ cup extra-virgin olive oil

1 garlic clove, minced

½ cup almonds, chopped

2 medium tomatoes, seeded and chopped

¼ cup fresh Italian parsley

2 tablespoons red wine vinegar

1 teaspoon paprika

½ teaspoon red pepper flakes

½ teaspoon sea salt

8 ounces whole-wheat angel-hair pasta, cooked according to package instructions and drained

1. In a blender or food processor, combine the red red peppers, olive oil, garlic, almonds, tomatoes, parsley, red wine vinegar, paprika, red pepper flakes, and salt. Process for 20 one-second pulses, until the texture is similar to pesto.

2. Toss with the hot pasta and serve.

Substitution tip: You can make this gluten-free by replacing the pasta with zucchini noodles or gluten-free pasta. Make it nut-free by replacing the almonds with an equal amount of pepitas.

Per Serving: Calories: 470; Total fat: 24g; Saturated fat: 3g; Cholesterol: 0mg; Carbohydrates: 54g; Fiber: 11g; Protein: 14g; Sodium: 300mg

SPAGHETTI WITH MUSHROOM AND PEPPER RAGOUT

VEGAN

Serves 4 | Prep time: 10 minutes | Cook time: 15 minutes | Serving size: 1 cup pasta and ½ cup sauce

This hearty and flavorful mushroom and pepper sauce is the perfect topping for spaghetti or your favorite pasta shape. The ragout has tender veggies and savory, earthy mushrooms that will fill you up. You can use the red wine in the sauce, and then drink a glass with dinner.

3 tablespoons extra-virgin olive oil

2 shallots, minced

1 pound cremini mushrooms, chopped

1 red bell pepper, seeded and chopped

1 teaspoon dried thyme

¼ teaspoon red pepper flakes

½ teaspoon sea salt

¼ teaspoon freshly ground black pepper

3 garlic cloves, minced

½ cup dry red wine

8 ounces whole-wheat spaghetti, cooked according to package instructions and drained

1. In a large pot, heat the olive oil over medium-high heat until it shimmers.
2. Add the shallots and cook until soft, about 3 minutes. Add the mushrooms, bell pepper, thyme, red pepper flakes, salt, and black pepper. Cook, stirring occasionally, until the mushrooms are browned, 5 to 7 minutes.
3. Add the garlic and cook, stirring constantly, for 30 seconds.
4. Pour the wine into the pot, using the side of a spoon to scrape any browned bits from the bottom of the pan. Simmer, stirring, until the wine is reduced by half, 2 to 3 minutes more.
5. Toss with the hot pasta and serve.

Substitution tip: You can make this gluten-free by replacing the pasta with zucchini noodles or gluten-free pasta.

Per Serving: Calories: 370; Total fat: 12g; Saturated fat: 2g; Cholesterol: 0mg; Carbohydrates: 50g; Fiber: 8g; Protein: 13g; Sodium: 299mg

PESTO PENNE

VEGETARIAN

Serves 4 | Prep time: 10 minutes | Serving size: 1 cup pasta and 2 tablespoons sauce

Pesto is a quick but flavorful uncooked sauce made with just a few simple ingredients. It's at its best when tender basil is in season in the spring and summer. Sometimes during the late spring or early summer, you can find garlic scapes at your local farmers' market, which make a delicious substitute for the garlic in pesto.

½ cup fresh basil

¼ cup pine nuts

2 garlic cloves, chopped

¼ cup extra-virgin olive oil

¼ cup grated
Parmesan cheese

Juice of ½ lemon

½ teaspoon sea salt

¼ teaspoon red
pepper flakes

8 ounces whole-wheat
penne pasta, cooked
according to package
instructions and drained

1. In a blender or food processor, combine the basil, pine nuts, garlic, olive oil, Parmesan cheese, lemon juice, and salt. Process for 20 one-second pulses, or until all the ingredients are finely chopped.
2. Toss with the hot pasta and serve.

Nutritional boost: Make this heart-healthier by replacing the pine nuts with walnuts and adding ½ cup of chopped kale or 1 cup of baby spinach.

Per Serving: Calories: 421; Total fat: 23g; Saturated fat: 4g; Cholesterol: 5mg; Carbohydrates: 44g; Fiber: 7g; Protein: 13g; Sodium: 408mg

VEGGIE PITA PIZZAS

VEGETARIAN

Serves 4 | Prep time: 10 minutes | Cook time: 10 minutes | Serving size: 1 pizza

Instead of traditional pizza sauce, these pizzas use the sauce from Pasta Romesco (page 90). It gives the pizzas extra flavor and serves as the perfect base for all kinds of vegetables and a sprinkling of cheese.

4 whole-wheat pitas

½ recipe romesco sauce

1 (14-ounce) can artichoke bottoms, drained and chopped

1 (4-ounce) can sliced black olives

½ red onion, minced

1 cup crumbled feta cheese

1. Preheat the oven to 425°F. Line a rimmed baking sheet with parchment paper.
2. Place the whole pitas on the prepared baking sheet. Spread them with the sauce.
3. Top with the artichoke bottoms, olives, and onion. Sprinkle with the feta cheese.
4. Bake until the cheese melts and bubbles, about 8 minutes. Serve.

Per Serving: Calories: 450; Total fat: 25g; Saturated fat: 7g; Cholesterol: 33mg; Carbohydrates: 44g; Fiber: 9g; Protein: 16g; Sodium: 1,151mg

COUSCOUS WITH ROASTED VEGGIES

VEGAN

Serves 4 | Prep time: 10 minutes | Cook time: 40 minutes
Serving size: 1 cup couscous and 1½ cups vegetables

These simple oven-roasted vegetables don't take much active time, but they do take about 40 minutes to develop deeply caramelized flavors in the oven. Delicious by themselves as a side dish, the veggies are even better served as a meal over quick-cooking couscous.

6 shallots, quartered

3 large carrots, peeled and sliced

2 fennel bulbs, cut into 1-inch cubes

1 butternut squash, seeded and chopped into 1-inch cubes

2 medium zucchini, cut into 1-inch cubes

2 red bell peppers, seeded and cut into large pieces

3 tablespoons extra-virgin olive oil

1 tablespoon chopped fresh rosemary

½ teaspoon sea salt

¼ teaspoon freshly ground black pepper

1 cup whole-wheat couscous, cooked according to package instructions

1. Preheat the oven to 475°F.
2. In a large bowl, combine the shallots, carrots, fennel, squash, zucchini, and bell peppers. Add the olive oil, rosemary, salt, and black pepper. Mix well.
3. Spread the mixture in a single layer on two large rimmed baking sheets.
4. Bake for about 40 minutes, or until the vegetables are browned and tender.
5. Spoon over the couscous and serve.

Substitution tip: Make this gluten-free by replacing the couscous with cooked quinoa.

Per Serving: Calories: 416; Total fat: 12g; Saturated fat: 2g; Cholesterol: 0mg; Carbohydrates: 75g; Fiber: 13g; Protein: 11g; Sodium: 414mg

MEDITERRANEAN-SPICED QUINOA-STUFFED EGGPLANT

ALLERGEN-FREE, GLUTEN-FREE, VEGAN

Serves 4 | Prep time: 10 minutes | Cook time: 1 hour | Serving size: ½ eggplant and 1 cup filling

Eggplant is a Mediterranean diet mainstay. An excellent source of fiber, vitamin B_1, and copper, eggplant may lower levels of "bad" cholesterol in your blood. When cooked, it literally melts in your mouth. That's why quinoa or any type of whole grain (barley, brown rice, farro) provides a nice contrast and texture to this savory and spicy favorite.

2 medium eggplants, all but about ½ inch of the flesh scooped out

2 tablespoons extra-virgin olive oil

1 onion, chopped

2 garlic cloves, minced

1 (15-ounce) can white beans, drained and rinsed

1 (15-ounce) can crushed tomatoes, drained

Zest and juice of 1 lemon, divided

1 teaspoon dried oregano

½ teaspoon sea salt

2 cups cooked quinoa

1. Preheat the oven to 350°F. Line a rimmed baking sheet with parchment paper.
2. Place the eggplant halves, cut-side up, on the prepared baking sheet.
3. In a large skillet, heat the olive oil over medium-high heat until it shimmers. Add the onion and cook until it softens, about 3 minutes.
4. Add the garlic and cook, stirring constantly, for 30 seconds.
5. Add the white beans, tomatoes, lemon zest, oregano, and salt. Cook, stirring, for 5 minutes.
6. Stir in the quinoa and lemon juice.
7. Spoon the mixture into the eggplant halves.
8. Bake until the eggplants are soft, about 50 minutes.

Nutritional boost: **Add crunch and some heart-healthy fats by sprinkling each stuffed eggplant with 2 tablespoons of almond flour before baking.**

Per Serving: Calories: 364; Total fat: 10g; Saturated fat: 1g; Cholesterol: 0mg; Carbohydrates: 63g; Fiber: 18g; Protein: 17g; Sodium: 669mg

COUSCOUS WITH WHITE BEANS AND GREENS

VEGAN

Serves 4 | Prep time: 10 minutes | Cook time: 15 minutes | Serving size: 1 cup couscous and 1 cup sauce

This is another quick stir-fry that's spicy and flavorful. When you serve it on top of fluffy, orange-scented couscous, it's truly a delicious meal you'll crave.

¾ cup freshly squeezed orange juice, divided

½ cup water

1 cup whole-wheat instant couscous

2 tablespoons extra-virgin olive oil

1 red onion, chopped

1 red bell pepper, seeded and chopped

1 garlic clove, minced

1 (15-ounce) can white beans, drained and rinsed

1 pint grape tomatoes, halved

1 teaspoon dried oregano

½ teaspoon sea salt

2 cups baby spinach

1. In a medium saucepan, combine ½ cup of orange juice and the water. Bring to a boil over medium-high heat.

2. Remove from the heat. Stir in the couscous. Cover and allow to sit for 10 minutes.

3. While the couscous rests, in a large skillet, heat the olive oil over medium-high heat until it shimmers.

4. Add the onion and bell pepper and cook, stirring occasionally, until the vegetables are soft, about 4 minutes.

5. Add the garlic and cook, stirring constantly, for 30 seconds.

6. Add the beans, tomatoes, oregano, and salt. Cook, stirring, for 4 minutes. Add the spinach and cook, stirring, for 1 minute. Add the remaining ¼ cup of orange juice. Cook for 1 minute more.

7. Fluff the couscous with a fork. Spoon the sauce over the couscous and serve.

Nutritional boost: Add heart-healthy antioxidants by garnishing this dish with 2 tablespoons of pomegranate seeds per serving.

Per Serving: Calories: 353; Total fat: 8g; Saturated fat: 1g; Cholesterol: 0mg; Carbohydrates: 63g; Fiber: 9g; Protein: 14g; Sodium: 557mg

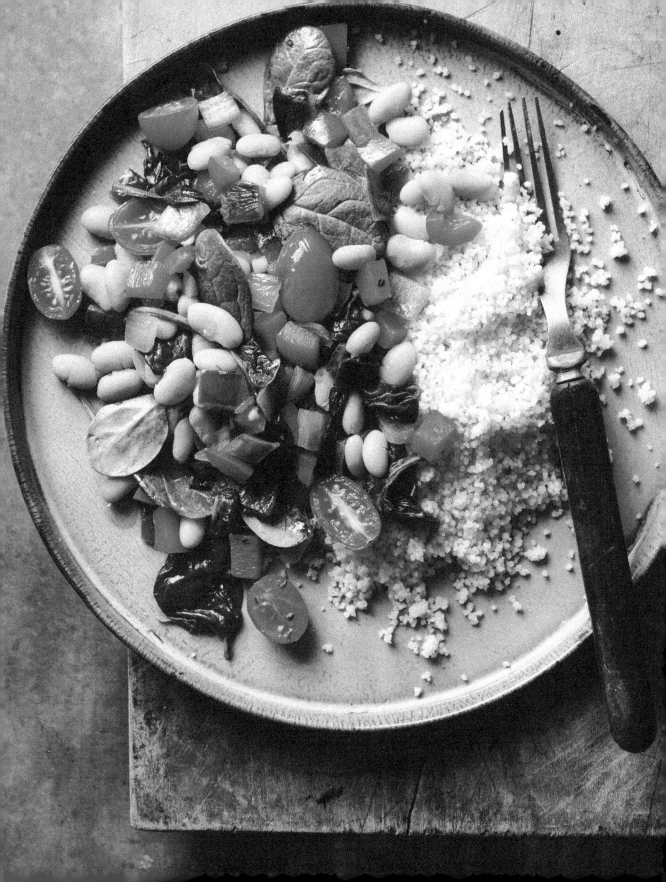

ZUCCHINI FRITTERS WITH RED PEPPER SAUCE

GLUTEN-FREE, VEGETARIAN

Serves 6 | Prep time: 10 minutes | Cook time: 20 minutes | Serving size: 2 fritters

Deep-fried zucchini fritters? No way! These enticing fritters are perfectly seasoned and pair beautifully with a creamy roasted red pepper sauce to make a delicious vegetarian main. You can also have them for breakfast in place of hash browns.

2 medium zucchini, grated on a box grater

½ red onion, grated

1 red bell pepper, seeded and very finely chopped or grated

1 garlic clove, minced

1 egg, beaten

½ cup almond flour

¼ cup chopped fresh dill

¾ teaspoon sea salt, divided

¼ teaspoon freshly ground black pepper

1 (12-ounce) jar roasted red peppers, drained

½ cup nonfat plain Greek yogurt

1. Preheat the oven to 400°F. Line two large baking sheets with parchment paper and set aside.
2. Wrap the grated zucchini and onion in a tea towel or paper towel. Wring over the sink to squeeze out as much moisture as possible. Put into a large bowl.
3. Add the bell pepper, garlic, egg, almond flour, dill, ½ teaspoon of salt, and the black pepper. Mix well.
4. Form the mixture into 12 balls and place them on the prepared baking sheets. Flatten with a plate or spatula.
5. Bake for 20 minutes, or until browned, flipping halfway through.
6. While the fritters bake, in a blender or food processor, combine the roasted red peppers, Greek yogurt, and the remaining ¼ teaspoon of salt. Blend until smooth.
7. Serve the fritters with the sauce spooned on top.

Variation tip: Replace the grated zucchini with 2 peeled, grated sweet potatoes. You'll still need to squeeze the water out of the onions, but not the potatoes.

Per Serving: Calories: 111; Total fat: 6g; Saturated fat: 1g; Cholesterol: 31mg; Carbohydrates: 11g; Fiber: 3g; Protein: 7g; Sodium: 319mg

FETA AND SPINACH STUFFED PORTOBELLO MUSHROOMS

GLUTEN-FREE, VEGETARIAN

Serves 4 | Prep time: 15 minutes | Cook time: 1 hour | Serving size: 1 mushroom and ½ cup filling

Stuffed with savory herbed spinach and feta cheese, portobello mushrooms make the perfect vessel for a nutritious and tasty meal. If you want to reduce cooking time to only 10 minutes, you can also stuff smaller cremini mushrooms.

4 portobello mushrooms

2 tablespoons extra-virgin olive oil, divided

1 red onion, chopped

1 tablespoon dried Italian seasoning

6 cups baby spinach

½ (12-ounce) jar roasted red peppers, drained and chopped

½ teaspoon sea salt

3 garlic cloves, minced

¼ cup pine nuts

1 cup cooked brown rice

½ cup crumbled feta cheese

1. Preheat the oven to 375°F. Line a baking sheet with parchment paper.
2. Use a spoon to remove the stems and black gills from the mushrooms. Place them, cavity-side up, on the prepared baking sheet.
3. In a large skillet, heat the olive oil over medium-high heat until it shimmers. Add the onion and Italian seasoning and cook until the onions are soft, about 4 minutes.
4. Add the spinach, roasted red peppers, and salt. Cook, stirring, until the spinach is soft, about 2 minutes more. Add the garlic and cook, stirring constantly, for 30 seconds.
5. Remove from the heat. Stir in the pine nuts and rice.
6. Spoon the mixture into the mushroom caps and sprinkle the feta cheese on top.
7. Bake until the mushrooms are tender, about 50 minutes. Serve.

Ingredient tip: Don't run mushrooms under water to clean them—it waterlogs them because mushrooms are super absorbent. Instead, use a paper towel or a mushroom brush to gently wipe away any visible dirt.

Per Serving: Calories: 290; Total fat: 19g; Saturated fat: 5g; Cholesterol: 17mg; Carbohydrates: 25g; Fiber: 5g; Protein: 8g; Sodium: 560mg

SWEET POTATO PUREE WITH CREAMY MUSHROOM SAUCE

VEGETARIAN

Serves 4 | Prep time: 15 minutes | Cook time: 15 minutes
Serving size: ½ cup potatoes and ½ cup sauce

The earthy flavor of mushrooms is a lovely complement to the sweetness of sweet potatoes, and their meaty texture contrasts nicely with the smooth potatoes. This is essentially an elevated vegetarian version of potatoes and gravy, but it's really tasty.

3 sweet potatoes, peeled and cut into ½-inch cubes

2 tablespoons extra-virgin olive oil

1 shallot, minced

8 ounces button mushrooms, sliced

1 teaspoon dried thyme

3 garlic cloves, minced

2 tablespoons whole-wheat flour

3 cups low-sodium vegetable broth

1 teaspoon sea salt, divided

½ teaspoon freshly ground black pepper, divided

¼ cup nonfat plain Greek yogurt

¼ cup skim milk

1. Put the potatoes in a large pot and cover with water by at least 2 inches. Place over high heat and bring to a boil. Cover and continue boiling until the potatoes are fork-tender, about 10 minutes.

2. While the potatoes cook, in a large skillet, heat the olive oil over medium-high heat until it shimmers.

3. Add the shallot, mushrooms, and thyme and cook, stirring occasionally, until the mushrooms are browned, 5 to 7 minutes.

4. Add the garlic and cook, stirring constantly, for 30 seconds.

5. Add the flour and cook, stirring, for 1 minute.

6. Pour the broth into the skillet and stir until it boils and thickens, about 3 minutes. Season with the remaining ½ teaspoon of salt and ¼ teaspoon of pepper.

7. Once the potatoes are cooked, drain them and return them to the pot. Add the yogurt, milk, remaining ½ teaspoon of salt, and remaining ¼ teaspoon of pepper. Use a hand mixer or immersion blender to blend until smooth. Alternatively, you can mash the sweet potatoes by themselves with a potato masher and then stir in the yogurt, milk, salt, and pepper.

8. Serve the sweet potatoes with the mushroom sauce spooned over them.

Per Serving: Calories: 220; Total fat: 8g; Saturated fat: 1g; Cholesterol: <1mg; Carbohydrates: 34g; Fiber: 5g; Protein: 6g; Sodium: 715mg

ROASTED EGGPLANT WITH GARLIC SAUCE

VEGETARIAN

Serves 4 | Prep time: 25 minutes | Cook time: 5 minutes
Serving size: ¼ eggplant and 2 tablespoons sauce

If you like garlic, chances are you'll love this Lebanese-inspired sauce. Here, it adds a bold lemon-garlic punch of flavor to simple roasted eggplant.

2 medium eggplants, cut into ½-inch slices

2 teaspoons sea salt, divided

10 garlic cloves, smashed

¼ cup extra-virgin olive oil, plus 1 tablespoon

Juice of 1 lemon

¼ teaspoon ground cinnamon

⅛ teaspoon freshly ground black pepper

⅛ teaspoon ground cumin

⅛ teaspoon ground nutmeg

⅛ teaspoon ground coriander

1. Put the eggplant slices in a colander over a bowl or in the sink. Sprinkle them with 1½ teaspoons of salt and let them drain for 20 minutes. Wipe away the salt and pat the eggplant slices dry.

2. While it drains, in a blender or food processor, combine the garlic and the remaining ½ teaspoon of salt. Process until finely chopped.

3. With the blender or food processor still running, pour in ¼ cup of olive oil in a thin stream until fully incorporated, then add the lemon juice and continue processing until mixed.

4. Preheat the oven's broiler to high.

5. Add the eggplant to a rimmed baking sheet. Brush the eggplant slices with the remaining 1 tablespoon of olive oil.

6. In a small bowl, mix together the cinnamon, pepper, cumin, nutmeg, and coriander. Sprinkle over the eggplant.

7. Broil until browned, about 2 minutes. Flip and broil for another 2 minutes.

8. Spoon the sauce on the slices and serve.

Ingredient tip: Peel garlic cloves quickly and easily by first smashing them with a meat-tenderizing mallet.

Per Serving: Calories: 237; Total fat: 18g; Saturated fat: 3g; Cholesterol: 0mg; Carbohydrates: 21g; Fiber: 7g; Protein: 3g; Sodium: 1,172mg

HEARTY SAGE, SQUASH, AND CHICKPEA STEW

VEGAN

Serves 6 | Prep time: 10 minutes | Cook time: 20 minutes | Serving size: 1½ cups

Squash and sage have a natural affinity for each other, and this quick and hearty stew capitalizes on that delicious flavor combination. Fiber-rich chickpeas help you feel fuller longer and add a buttery and nutty bite.

2 tablespoons extra-virgin olive oil

1 onion, finely chopped

3 cups cubed butternut squash (½-inch cubes)

2 teaspoons ground sage

3 garlic cloves, minced

2 tablespoons whole-wheat flour

2 cups low-sodium vegetable broth

1 (15-ounce) can chickpeas, drained and rinsed

½ teaspoon sea salt

¼ teaspoon freshly ground black pepper

1. In a large pot, heat the olive oil over medium-high heat until it shimmers.
2. Add the onion, squash, and sage and cook, stirring occasionally, until the squash is tender, about 15 minutes.
3. Add the garlic and cook, stirring constantly, for 30 seconds.
4. Add the flour and cook, stirring, for 1 minute.
5. Add the broth and use the side of a spoon to scrape any browned bits from the bottom of the pot. Add the chickpeas, salt, and pepper. Cook, stirring occasionally, until the stew thickens and the chickpeas are warmed, 3 to 4 minutes. Serve.

Per Serving: Calories: 174; Total fat: 5g; Saturated fat: 1g; Cholesterol: 0mg; Carbohydrates: 29g; Fiber: 7g; Protein: 5g; Sodium: 328mg

EASY VEGAN PAELLA

ALLERGEN-FREE, GLUTEN-FREE, VEGAN

Serves 6 | Prep time: 10 minutes, plus 10 minutes to sit | Cook time: 30 minutes | Serving size: 1 cup

Paella, a well-known rice dish in Spanish cuisine, takes on an enticing golden color thanks to saffron, which is considered the world's most expensive spice. This recipe needs only a few threads, so buy saffron in very small amounts. It's well worth the unforgettable, extremely subtle, slightly sweet, and luxuriously fragrant flavor it adds to this dish.

4 cups low-sodium vegetable broth

½ teaspoon saffron threads

2 tablespoons extra-virgin olive oil

1 onion, finely diced

1 red bell pepper, seeded and finely diced

4 garlic cloves, minced

1 roma tomato, seeded and diced

1½ teaspoons paprika

1 teaspoon dried thyme

½ teaspoon sea salt

1½ cups Arborio (risotto) rice

½ cup fresh or frozen peas (thawed if frozen)

1. In a small pot, bring the broth to a boil. Reduce the heat to medium-low and add the saffron threads. Simmer for 1 minute. Keep warm on low heat while you prepare the rice.

2. In a large skillet, heat the olive oil over medium-high heat until it shimmers.

3. Add the onion and bell pepper and cook until the vegetables begin to brown, 3 to 4 minutes.

4. Add the garlic and cook, stirring constantly, for 30 seconds.

5. Add the tomato, paprika, thyme, and salt. Cook, stirring, for 3 minutes more.

6. Spread the rice in an even layer in the skillet and carefully pour in the warm broth. Do not stir.

7. Reduce the heat to medium-low. Simmer without stirring until the liquid is absorbed, about 20 minutes.

8. Remove from the heat. Add the peas over the top of the rice and cover the skillet with foil or a plate. Allow the paella to sit for 10 minutes before serving.

Ingredient tip: If you can't find saffron (or if it's too expensive), you can replace it with ½ teaspoon of turmeric.

Per Serving: Calories: 243; Total fat: 5g; Saturated fat: 1g; Cholesterol: 0mg; Carbohydrates: 45g; Fiber: 3g; Protein: 4g; Sodium: 303mg

SAVORY CHICKPEA AND VEGGIE SAUTÉ

ALLERGEN-FREE, GLUTEN-FREE, VEGAN

Serves 4 | Prep time: 10 minutes | Cook time: 10 minutes | Serving size: 1½ cups

If you need a meal fast, then stir-frying is always your best bet. And there's no reason why a stir-fry can't have Mediterranean flavors instead of Asian. You'll have this fragrant and delicious sauté on your table in less than 20 minutes.

3 tablespoons extra-virgin olive oil

1 red onion, chopped

1 red bell pepper, seeded and chopped

½ cup sun-dried tomatoes, drained and chopped

1 zucchini, chopped

1 (15-ounce) can artichoke bottoms, drained and chopped

1 (15-ounce) can chickpeas, drained and rinsed

1 tablespoon dried Italian seasoning

2 cups baby spinach

3 garlic cloves, minced

Juice of 1 lemon

1. In a large skillet, heat the olive oil over medium-high heat until it shimmers.
2. Add the onion, bell pepper, tomatoes, zucchini, artichoke bottoms, chickpeas, and Italian seasoning. Cook, stirring, until the onions soften, about 5 minutes.
3. Add the spinach and cook, stirring, for another 2 minutes.
4. Add the garlic and cook, stirring constantly, for 30 seconds.
5. Add the lemon juice. Cook until it evaporates, about 1 minute more. Serve immediately.

Ingredient tip: To help the artichoke bottoms and sun-dried tomatoes brown well, pat them dry with a paper towel before you add them.

Per Serving: Calories: 304; Total fat: 15g; Saturated fat: 2g; Cholesterol: 0mg; Carbohydrates: 36g; Fiber: 11g; Protein: 9g; Sodium: 537mg

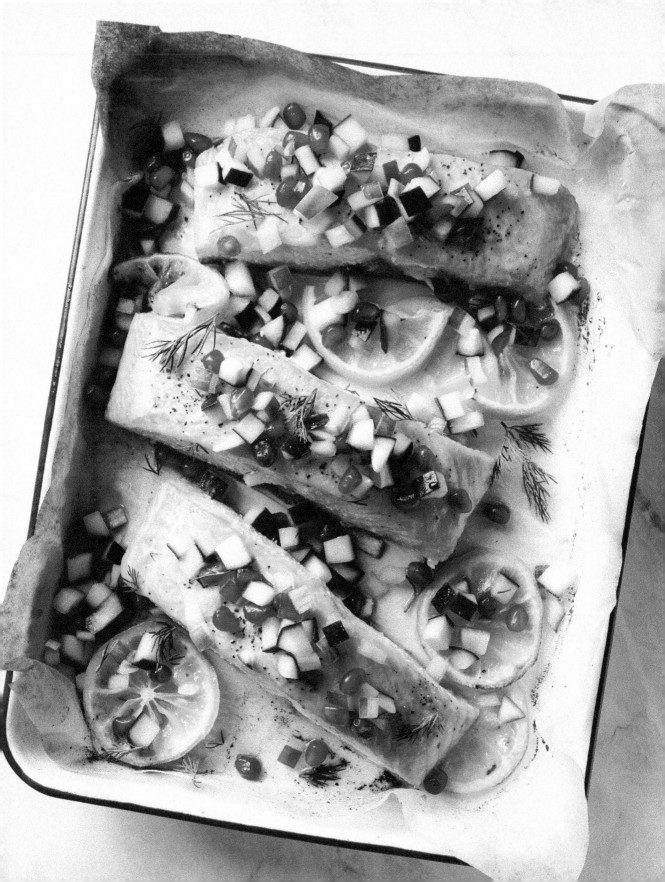

SEAFOOD ENTRÉES

< *Salmon with Pomegranate Salsa,*
page 122

PAN-SEARED SCALLOPS WITH TOMATO AND WINE-BRAISED KALE

GLUTEN-FREE

Serves 4 | Prep time: 10 minutes | Cook time: 15 minutes
Serving size: About 6 scallops and ½ cup kale

A fancy, rich, and savory dish, this recipe looks like a million bucks when served to family or friends. Kale's dark, leafy greens mean loads of fiber, potassium, and vitamin C, all good for reducing blood pressure. Even better, it's a hearty meal that satisfies cravings yet is easy on the waistline.

3 tablespoons extra-virgin olive oil, divided

3 garlic cloves, minced

1 (14-ounce) can chopped tomatoes, drained

½ cup dry white wine

4 cups chopped kale

1 teaspoon sea salt, divided

¼ teaspoon freshly ground black pepper, divided

¼ teaspoon red pepper flakes

1 pound sea scallops

1. In a large pot, heat 1 tablespoon of olive oil over medium-high heat until it shimmers.

2. Add the garlic and cook, stirring constantly, for 30 seconds.

3. Add the tomatoes and white wine and bring to a simmer. Add the kale, ½ teaspoon of salt, ⅛ teaspoon of black pepper, and the red pepper flakes. Stir to mix and cook, covered, until the kale is soft, about 5 minutes.

4. Uncover and simmer another 2 to 3 minutes to allow most of the liquid to evaporate.

5. While the kale cooks, trim the small muscular attachment from the side of each scallop and discard. Rinse the scallops in a colander and pat dry. Season with the remaining ½ teaspoon of salt and remaining ⅛ teaspoon of black pepper.

6. In a large nonstick skillet, heat the remaining 2 tablespoons of olive oil over medium-high heat until it shimmers.

7. Add the scallops and cook without disturbing them until browned on the bottom, 2 to 3 minutes. Flip and cook on the other side until browned, about 2 minutes more.

8. Serve the kale with the scallops on top of it.

Variation tip: You can also use an equal amount of Swiss chard to replace the kale in this recipe.

Per Serving: Calories: 278; Total fat: 12g; Saturated fat: 2g; Cholesterol: 37mg; Carbohydrates: 18g; Fiber: 4g; Protein: 23g; Sodium: 931mg

SHRIMP SCAMPI

Serves 4 | **Prep time: 10 minutes** | **Cook time: 10 minutes** | Serving size: 1 cup pasta and 1 cup shrimp

A classic recipe using heart-healthy olive oil, shrimp scampi goes perfectly with whole-grain pasta. The trick with shrimp scampi is to avoid overcooking, which causes a rubbery texture—once you add the shrimp to the pan, cook just until they turn pink all over.

3 tablespoons extra-virgin olive oil

1 shallot, finely chopped

1 pound medium shrimp, peeled and deveined

4 garlic cloves, minced

½ cup dry white wine

½ teaspoon sea salt

¼ teaspoon freshly ground black pepper

¼ teaspoon red pepper flakes

8 ounces whole-wheat or gluten-free spaghetti, cooked according to package instructions and drained

¼ cup chopped fresh basil

1. In a large skillet, heat the olive oil over medium-high heat until it shimmers.
2. Add the shallot and cook, stirring occasionally, until soft, about 3 minutes.
3. Add the shrimp and cook, stirring, just until pink, 3 to 4 minutes.
4. Add the garlic and cook, stirring constantly, for 30 seconds.
5. Add the wine, salt, black pepper, and red pepper flakes. Bring to a simmer and cook until the wine is reduced by half, about 3 minutes more.
6. Toss with the spaghetti. Sprinkle with the basil before serving.

Nutritional boost: Substituting salmon for the shrimp adds beneficial heart-healthy omega-3 fatty acids. Use 1 pound of fish, cut into 1-inch pieces, in place of the shrimp.

Per Serving: Calories: 379; Total fat: 14g; Saturated fat: 2g; Cholesterol: 145mg; Carbohydrates: 44g; Fiber: 6g; Protein: 24g; Sodium: 408mg

GARLIC-LEMON SHRIMP AND RICE SKILLET

GLUTEN-FREE

Serves 4 | **Prep time: 15 minutes** | **Cook time: 15 minutes** | **Serving size: ¾ cup**

You can have this dish as a simple dinner on a weekday even though it's impressive enough to serve guests at a dinner party. Complete the meal by serving with an antioxidant-rich salad mix of leafy greens and a glass of red wine, if desired.

3 tablespoons extra-virgin olive oil

1 onion, chopped

1 red bell pepper, seeded and chopped

1 pound medium shrimp, peeled and deveined

4 garlic cloves, minced

Juice of 3 lemons

1 tablespoon dried Italian seasoning

½ teaspoon sea salt

¼ teaspoon freshly ground black pepper

¼ teaspoon red pepper flakes

1 cup cooked brown rice

1. In a large skillet, heat the olive oil over medium-high heat until it shimmers.
2. Add the onion and bell pepper and cook, stirring occasionally, until soft, about 4 minutes.
3. Add the shrimp and cook, stirring, just until pink, 3 to 4 minutes.
4. Add the garlic and cook, stirring constantly, for 30 seconds.
5. Add the lemon juice, Italian seasoning, salt, black pepper, and red pepper flakes. Bring to a simmer and cook until the liquid is reduced by half, about 2 minutes.
6. Stir in the rice. Cook, stirring, until the rice warms through, about 2 minutes more. Serve.

Substitution tip: If you have a shellfish allergy but not a fish allergy, you can substitute 1 pound of chopped cod or salmon for the shrimp.

Per Serving: Calories: 260; Total fat: 12g; Saturated fat: 2g; Cholesterol: 145mg; Carbohydrates: 21g; Fiber: 3g; Protein: 20g; Sodium: 408mg

PRAWN AND ORZO STEW

Serves 4 | **Prep time: 15 minutes** | **Cook time: 20 minutes** | **Serving size: 1 cup**

Not to be mistaken for shrimp—they're not the same thing—prawns are a popular seafood around the world. Of course, lovers of shrimp can use them instead. This stew is a spicy blend of scrumptious, mesmerizing flavors.

2 tablespoons extra-virgin olive oil

1 onion, chopped

2 carrots, peeled and chopped

1 fennel bulb, chopped

1 pound medium prawns, peeled and deveined

3 garlic cloves, minced

1 (14-ounce) can crushed tomatoes

1 tablespoon dried Italian seasoning

1 cup chopped black olives

½ teaspoon sea salt

¼ teaspoon freshly ground black pepper

1 cup whole-wheat orzo, cooked according to package instructions and drained

1. In a large pot, heat the olive oil over medium-high heat until it shimmers.
2. Add the onion, carrots, and fennel and cook, stirring occasionally, until the veggies begin to brown, about 5 minutes.
3. Add the prawns and cook, stirring, just until pink, 3 to 4 minutes.
4. Add the garlic and cook, stirring constantly, for 30 seconds.
5. Add the tomatoes with their juices, Italian seasoning, olives, salt, and pepper. Bring to a simmer and cook, stirring occasionally, for 5 minutes.
6. Stir in the orzo. Cook until warmed through, another 1 to 2 minutes. Serve.

Ingredient tip: If you like, garnish this with ½ cup of chopped sun-dried tomatoes. If you prefer a spicier stew, you can add red pepper flakes to taste in step 5.

Per Serving: Calories: 455; Total fat: 13g; Saturated fat: 1g; Cholesterol: 260mg; Carbohydrates: 47g; Fiber: 6g; Protein: 38g; Sodium: 946mg

LEMON ORZO WITH ALBACORE TUNA AND PEAS

Serves 4 | Prep time: 15 minutes | Cook time: 15 minutes | Serving size: 1 cup

One of my favorite mixtures is tuna and peas. Both are delicious and highly nutritious for heart health, a total win-win. Add in a lemony base along with whole-wheat orzo, and your heart will thank you for this easy meal.

2 tablespoons extra-virgin olive oil

1 onion, chopped

1 red bell pepper, seeded and chopped

2 (5-ounce) cans albacore tuna, drained

2 garlic cloves, minced

Juice of 3 lemons

1 cup fresh or frozen peas

½ teaspoon sea salt

¼ teaspoon freshly ground black pepper

1 cup whole-wheat orzo, cooked according to package instructions and drained

¼ cup chopped fresh basil

1. In a large skillet, heat the olive oil over medium-high heat until it shimmers.
2. Add the onion and bell pepper and cook, stirring occasionally, until the vegetables are soft, about 4 minutes.
3. Add the tuna and cook, stirring, for 2 minutes.
4. Add the garlic and cook, stirring constantly, for 30 seconds.
5. Add the lemon juice, peas, salt, and black pepper. Bring to a simmer and cook until the liquid is reduced by half, about 3 minutes more.
6. Stir in the orzo. Cook until warmed through, another 1 to 2 minutes.
7. Garnish with the chopped fresh basil and serve.

Substitution tip: Make this gluten-free by replacing the orzo with 2 cups of cooked quinoa.

Per Serving: Calories: 347; Total fat: 9g; Saturated fat: 1g; Cholesterol: 25mg; Carbohydrates: 44g; Fiber: 4g; Protein: 24g; Sodium: 368mg

ALBACORE TUNA AND TOMATO ROTINI

Serves 4 | Prep time: 15 minutes | Cook time: 10 minutes | Serving size: 1½ cups

Blessed with essential omega-3 fatty acids, albacore tuna should be on your list of foods for heart health. Your taste buds will be in for a treat with the aromatic blend of fresh fennel, thick tomatoes, and earthy oregano and thyme, making this a captivating yet simple meal.

2 tablespoons extra-virgin olive oil

1 onion, chopped

1 red bell pepper, seeded and chopped

1 fennel bulb, chopped

2 (5-ounce) cans albacore tuna, drained

3 garlic cloves, minced

1 (15-ounce) can crushed tomatoes

1 (15-ounce) can white beans, drained and rinsed

1 teaspoon dried Italian seasoning

½ teaspoon sea salt

⅛ teaspoon freshly ground black pepper

1 cup whole-wheat rotini pasta, cooked according to package instructions and drained

1. In a large skillet, heat the olive oil over medium-high heat until it shimmers.
2. Add the onion, bell pepper, and fennel and cook, stirring occasionally, until the vegetables are soft, about 4 minutes.
3. Add the tuna and cook, stirring, for 2 minutes.
4. Add the garlic and cook, stirring constantly, for 30 seconds.
5. Add the tomatoes with their juices, white beans, Italian seasoning, salt, and black pepper. Cook, stirring occasionally, for 4 minutes.
6. Toss with the warm pasta and serve.

Per Serving: Calories: 347; Total fat: 10g; Saturated fat: 1g; Cholesterol: 25mg; Carbohydrates: 42g; Fiber: 10g; Protein: 29g; Sodium: 524mg

PARCHMENT-BAKED COD WITH ZUCCHINI AND TOMATOES

GLUTEN-FREE

Serves 4 | Prep time: 15 minutes | Cook time: 15 minutes | Serving size: 1 packet

A very easy, appetizing, and impressive dish, baked cod is perfect for anyone unsure of cooking fresh fish. This mild-flavored white fish is also a good source of omega-3 fatty acids and is rich in vitamins B_{12} and niacin as well as vitamins A, C, and E. Serve with a whole grain and fresh fruit to complement this meal.

4 (4-ounce) cod fillets

½ teaspoon sea salt

¼ teaspoon freshly ground black pepper

4 dill sprigs or 4 tablespoons chopped fresh dill

2 medium zucchini, chopped

1 cup cherry tomatoes, halved

8 slices lemon

2 tablespoons extra-virgin olive oil

1 cup dry white wine or low-sodium chicken broth

1. Preheat the oven to 400°F.
2. Lay out four pieces of parchment paper. Place 1 cod fillet in the center of each piece. Sprinkle the fillets with the salt and pepper. Place 1 dill sprig on each.
3. Fold up the sides of the parchment paper, leaving it open at the top. Transfer the packets to a rimmed baking sheet.
4. Divide the zucchini and tomatoes among the fillets, followed by the lemon slices. Drizzle each with ½ tablespoon of olive oil.
5. Carefully pour ¼ cup of wine into each packet and seal it by folding at the top.
6. Bake until the fillets are tender and flaky, about 15 minutes. Serve this meal in the packets.

Substitution tip: If you're allergic to fish but not shellfish, you can replace the cod with 4-ounce servings of sea scallops.

Per Serving: Calories: 248; Total fat: 8g; Saturated fat: 1g; Cholesterol: 62mg; Carbohydrates: 8g; Fiber: 3g; Protein: 27g; Sodium: 396mg

BRAISED WHITE FISH WITH CHICKPEAS AND RED PEPPERS

GLUTEN-FREE

Serves 4 | Prep time: 15 minutes | Cook time: 30 minutes
Serving size: 1 cod fillet and 1 cup vegetables

Here's another super-simple meal that comes together in no time. Use cod or any other white fish, such as halibut, to get the heart-healthy benefits of their omega-3 fat profile while enjoying chewy bites of vitamin C–rich red peppers and fiber-loaded chickpeas.

2 tablespoons extra-virgin olive oil

1 onion, chopped

1 red bell pepper, seeded and chopped

1 fennel bulb, thinly sliced

3 garlic cloves, minced

½ cup dry white wine or low-sodium chicken broth

1 (15-ounce) can crushed tomatoes

1 (15-ounce) can chickpeas, drained and rinsed

½ teaspoon sea salt

¼ teaspoon freshly ground black pepper

4 (4-ounce) cod fillets or another white fish

1. In a large, deep skillet or pot, heat the olive oil over medium-high heat until it shimmers.
2. And the onion, bell pepper, and fennel and cook, stirring occasionally, until the vegetables soften and begin to brown, about 7 minutes.
3. Add the garlic and cook, stirring constantly, for 30 seconds.
4. Add the wine, tomatoes with their juices, chickpeas, salt, and black pepper. Simmer for 10 minutes, stirring occasionally.
5. Add the fish, covering it with as much sauce as possible. Bring to a simmer and reduce the heat to medium-low. Cover and simmer until the fish is tender, 8 to 10 minutes more.
6. Serve the fish with the braising liquid and veggies spooned on top.

Ingredient tip: Add brightness and flavor by garnishing with ¼ cup of chopped fresh basil.

Per Serving: Calories: 359; Total fat: 9g; Saturated fat: 1g; Cholesterol: 62mg; Carbohydrates: 32g; Fiber: 9g; Protein: 35g; Sodium: 666mg

LEMON PEPPER COD

GLUTEN-FREE

Serves 4 | Prep time: 5 minutes | Cook time: 10 minutes | Serving size: 1 cod fillet

If dinner needs to be made quickly, this recipe is your answer. Within 15 minutes, you'll have this meal on the table ready to enjoy. Fresh lemon and dill reduce the need for excessive salt while making this meal pop with flavor.

4 (4-ounce) cod fillets

½ teaspoon sea salt

½ teaspoon freshly ground black pepper

Zest of 1 lemon and juice of 2 lemons, divided

2 tablespoons extra-virgin olive oil

1 tablespoon chopped fresh dill

1. Season the cod fillets with the salt, pepper, and lemon zest.

2. In a large nonstick skillet, heat the olive oil over medium-high heat until it shimmers.

3. Add the cod. Cook, undisturbed, until the cod releases easily from the pan, about 3 minutes.

4. Flip the cod. Add the lemon juice. Cook until the cod is cooked through, another 3 to 4 minutes.

5. Serve garnished with the dill.

Variation tip: You can also make cod scaloppine. Add 2 tablespoons of capers when you add the lemon juice. Remove the cod from the pan when it's cooked, but leave the pan on the heat and whisk in 2 tablespoons of very cold butter with any liquid that remains. Spoon the sauce over the cod and garnish with the dill.

Per Serving: Calories: 185; Total fat: 8g; Saturated fat: 1g; Cholesterol: 62mg; Carbohydrates: 2g; Fiber: <1g; Protein: 25g; Sodium: 379mg

TOMATO-POACHED COD

GLUTEN-FREE

Serves 4 | Prep time: 10 minutes | Cook time: 20 minutes | Serving size: 1 cod fillet and ½ cup sauce

Saucy, savory, and spicy—mild-flavored cod has never tasted so good. Serve with brown rice or couscous along with nutrient-dense roasted broccoli or Brussels sprouts, and you'll be feeding your heart just what the doctor ordered.

2 tablespoons extra-virgin olive oil

1 shallot, finely minced

2 garlic cloves, minced

1 (15-ounce) can chopped tomatoes

½ teaspoon ground cinnamon

¼ teaspoon ground allspice

½ teaspoon ground cumin

½ teaspoon ground coriander

½ teaspoon sea salt

¼ teaspoon freshly ground black pepper

4 (4-ounce) cod fillets

¼ cup chopped fresh cilantro

1. In a large, deep skillet or pot, heat the olive oil over medium-high heat until it shimmers.
2. Add the shallot and cook until soft, about 3 minutes.
3. Add the garlic and cook, stirring constantly, for 30 seconds.
4. Add the tomatoes with their juices, cinnamon, allspice, cumin, coriander, salt, and pepper. Stir.
5. Add the cod fillets and submerge them as much as possible in the sauce. Cover and simmer until the cod is white and flaky, about 15 minutes.
6. Sprinkle with the cilantro before serving.

Nutritional boost: Add heart-healthy fats and lots of flavor by adding ½ cup of sliced black olives to the recipe in step 4.

Per Serving: Calories: 207; Total fat: 8g; Saturated fat: 1g; Cholesterol: 62mg; Carbohydrates: 7g; Fiber: 2g; Protein: 27g; Sodium: 517mg

COD WITH MANGO SALSA

GLUTEN-FREE

Serves 4 | Prep time: 10 minutes | Cook time: 15 minutes | Serving size: 1 cod fillet and ¼ cup salsa

Who doesn't love a mango salsa? It's especially good with mild-flavored cod, which is a good source of blood-thinning omega-3 fats. Perfect for warm summer nights, this recipe is a refreshing dinner topped with a Mediterranean twist.

4 (4-ounce) cod fillets

2 tablespoons extra-virgin olive oil

1 teaspoon sea salt, divided

¼ teaspoon freshly ground black pepper

½ teaspoon ground cumin

4 slices lemon

2 mangos, peeled, pitted, and cubed

¼ red onion, finely minced

1 jalapeño pepper, seeded and finely chopped (optional)

¼ cup chopped fresh mint

Juice of ½ lemon

1. Preheat the oven to 400°F. Line a rimmed baking sheet with parchment paper.
2. Place the cod fillets on the prepared baking sheet and brush them with the olive oil. Sprinkle with ½ teaspoon of salt, the black pepper, and cumin. Place 1 lemon slice on each piece of cod.
3. Bake until the cod is tender, 10 to 15 minutes.
4. While the cod cooks, in a medium bowl, combine the mangos, onion, jalapeño pepper (if using), mint, lemon juice, and remaining ½ teaspoon of salt.
5. Serve the cod with the salsa spooned over the top.

Variation tip: If you can't find mangos, you can replace them with 1 cup of chopped cantaloupe, papaya, or pineapple.

Per Serving: Calories: 257; Total fat: 8g; Saturated fat: 1g; Cholesterol: 62mg; Carbohydrates: 21g; Fiber: 3g; Protein: 26g; Sodium: 675mg

HALIBUT WITH TOMATO AND OLIVE SALSA

GLUTEN-FREE

Serves 4 | Prep time: 10 minutes | Cook time: 15 minutes | Serving size: 1 halibut fillet and ¼ cup salsa

If you've never had halibut, you're in for a treat. Mild and delicately sweet, this white fish leaps with heart-healthy goodness—omega-3 fatty acids, niacin, selenium, and magnesium. And the salsa is colorful and bold, every bite capturing the essence of Mediterranean cuisine.

4 (4-ounce) halibut fillets

3 tablespoons extra-virgin olive oil, divided

1 teaspoon sea salt, divided

¼ teaspoon freshly ground black pepper

½ teaspoon ground oregano

2 large tomatoes, seeded and chopped

1 (4-ounce) can chopped black olives, drained

½ (12-ounce) jar roasted red peppers, drained

1 garlic clove, minced

¼ red onion, finely minced

Juice of ½ orange

2 tablespoons chopped fresh basil

1. Preheat the oven to 450°F. Line a rimmed baking sheet with parchment paper.
2. Place the halibut fillets on the prepared baking sheet and brush them with 1 tablespoon of olive oil. Sprinkle with ½ teaspoon of salt, the black pepper, and oregano.
3. Bake until the halibut is tender and flaky, 12 to 15 minutes.
4. While the halibut cooks, in a medium bowl, combine the tomatoes, olives, roasted red peppers, garlic, onion, orange juice, basil, remaining 2 tablespoons of olive oil, and remaining ½ teaspoon of salt.
5. Serve the halibut with the salsa spooned over the top.

Per Serving: Calories: 327; Total fat: 18g; Saturated fat: 2g; Cholesterol: 47mg; Carbohydrates: 9g; Fiber: 2g; Protein: 31g; Sodium: 845mg

BAKED SOLE WITH LEMON AND DILL

GLUTEN-FREE

Serves 4 | Prep time: 10 minutes | Cook time: 15 minutes | Serving size: 1 sole fillet

An easy-to-assemble sheet pan dish featuring delicate sole, this entrée will have everyone eagerly awaiting mealtime. Just add a side salad of baby spinach or kale with lots of fresh toppings and a slice of crusty whole-wheat bread with olive oil for dipping, and dinner is served.

4 (4-ounce) sole fillets

2 tablespoons extra-virgin olive oil

1 teaspoon garlic powder

1 teaspoon dried dill

½ teaspoon sea salt, divided

¼ teaspoon freshly ground black pepper

8 slices lemon

2 tablespoons capers, drained and rinsed

1. Preheat the oven to 375°F. Line a rimmed baking sheet with parchment paper.
2. Place the sole fillets on the prepared baking sheet.
3. In a small bowl, whisk together the olive oil, garlic powder, dill, salt, and pepper. Brush liberally on the sole. Top with the lemon slices and capers.
4. Bake until the sole is opaque and flaky, about 15 minutes. Serve.

Nutritional boost: Boost heart-healthy fats by adding almond flour (essentially crushed almonds) to the olive oil mixture in step 3; omit the lemon slices and capers.

Per Serving: Calories: 174; Total fat: 8g; Saturated fat: 2g; Cholesterol: 55mg; Carbohydrates: 4g; Fiber: 1g; Protein: 23g; Sodium: 456mg

SALMON WITH POMEGRANATE SALSA

GLUTEN-FREE

Serves 4 | Prep time: 10 minutes | Cook time: 15 minutes | Serving size: 1 salmon fillet and ½ cup salsa

Your search for a bold salsa is over. Tender, perfectly baked salmon fillets covered in a pomegranate salsa practically burst with zesty sweet and savory flavors everyone will love. Imagine how deliciously gorgeous this will look served with sautéed mixed greens and slices of heart-healthy avocado.

4 (4-ounce) salmon fillets

2 tablespoons extra-virgin olive oil

1 teaspoon sea salt, divided

¼ teaspoon freshly ground black pepper

4 slices lemon

½ cup pomegranate seeds

1 cucumber, chopped

¼ red onion, chopped

2 tablespoons chopped fresh dill

Juice of ½ lemon

1. Preheat the oven to 450°F.
2. Place the salmon fillets on a rimmed baking sheet. Brush with the olive oil and season with ½ teaspoon of salt and the pepper. Top each with a lemon slice.
3. Bake until the salmon is opaque and flaky, about 15 minutes.
4. While the salmon cooks, in a medium bowl, combine the pomegranate seeds, cucumber, onion, dill, lemon juice, and remaining ½ teaspoon of salt.
5. Serve the salmon topped with the salsa.

Nutritional boost: Add ¼ cup of chopped walnuts to the salsa to add texture and an additional boost of heart-healthy fats.

Per Serving: Calories: 237; Total fat: 12g; Saturated fat: 2g; Cholesterol: 85mg; Carbohydrates: 10g; Fiber: 3g; Protein: 24g; Sodium: 640mg

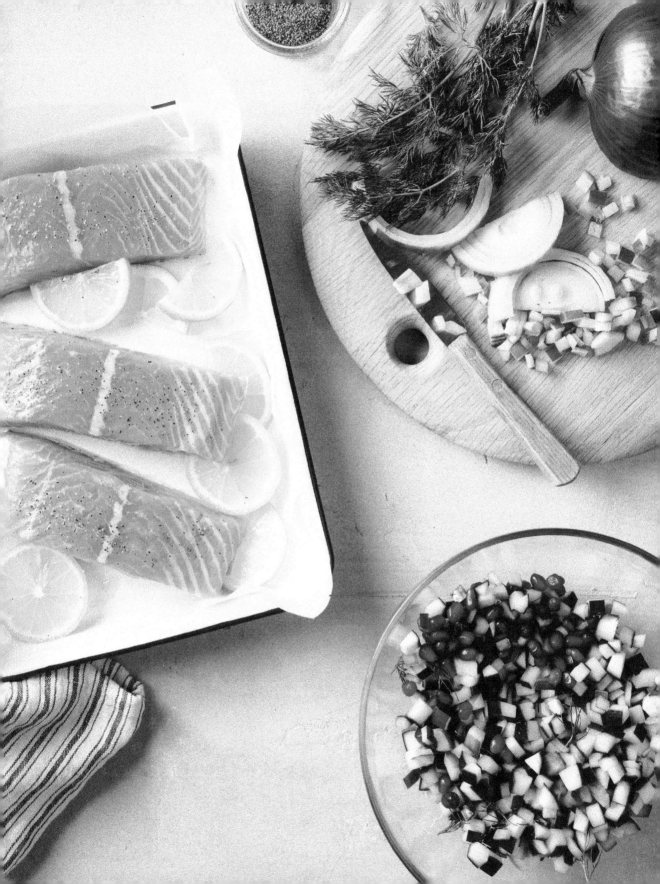

BALSAMIC-GLAZED SALMON

GLUTEN-FREE

Serves 4 | Prep time: 10 minutes | Cook time: 25 minutes | Serving size: 1 salmon fillet

No time to cook? No problem. Brushed with a sweet and lightly tangy balsamic glaze, this is a favorite way to prepare salmon, a staple of the Mediterranean diet. The end result is an amazingly delicious golden-brown fillet with a melt-in-your-mouth flavor.

2 tablespoons extra-virgin olive oil

1 shallot, finely minced

2 garlic cloves, minced

½ cup balsamic vinegar

¼ cup pure maple syrup

½ teaspoon sea salt

¼ teaspoon freshly ground black pepper

4 (4-ounce) salmon fillets

1. Preheat the oven to 450°F.
2. In a small saucepan, heat the olive oil over medium-high heat until it shimmers.
3. Add the shallot and cook, stirring occasionally, until soft, about 3 minutes.
4. Add the garlic and cook, stirring constantly, for 30 seconds.
5. Add the balsamic vinegar, maple syrup, salt, and pepper. Bring to a simmer. Simmer, stirring occasionally, until thick and syrupy, about 4 minutes more. Remove from the heat and let cool.
6. Place the salmon fillets on a rimmed baking sheet. Brush with the balsamic glaze.
7. Bake until the salmon is flaky, about 15 minutes.
8. While the salmon cooks, bring any leftover glaze to a boil. Reduce the heat to low and keep warm.
9. Spoon the reheated glaze over the salmon to serve.

Per Serving: Calories: 273; Total fat: 12g; Saturated fat: 2g; Cholesterol: 85mg; Carbohydrates: 19g; Fiber: 0g; Protein: 23g; Sodium: 358mg

ROASTED SALMON WITH FENNEL AND BELL PEPPER

GLUTEN-FREE

Serves 4 | **Prep time: 10 minutes** | **Cook time: 40 minutes**
Serving size: 1 salmon fillet and ½ cup vegetables

Fishing for a new salmon recipe? This one-pan delight features Mediterranean flavors, such as slightly sweet fennel and tangy citrus accents, for an outstanding meal that really shines. Serve straight from the oven to the table, making cleanup a breeze.

2 fennel bulbs, thinly sliced

1 red onion, thinly sliced

1 red bell pepper, seeded and thinly sliced

1 pint grape tomatoes, halved

2 tablespoons extra-olive olive oil

1 teaspoon sea salt, divided

½ teaspoon freshly ground black pepper, divided

1 teaspoon dried dill

1 (1-pound) center-cut salmon fillet

8 slices orange

1. Preheat the oven to 275°F.

2. In a large bowl, combine the fennel, onion, bell pepper, tomatoes, olive oil, ½ teaspoon of salt, ¼ teaspoon of black pepper, and the dill. Mix well.

3. Pour the mixture into a 9-by-13-inch baking dish. Place the salmon on top and season with the remaining ½ teaspoon of salt and ¼ teaspoon of black pepper. Arrange the orange slices on top of the salmon.

4. Bake until the salmon is opaque and flaky, about 35 to 40 minutes. Serve.

Variation tip: This works well with any center-cut fish fillet, such as trout or halibut.

Per Serving: Calories: 328; Total fat: 17g; Saturated fat: 4g; Cholesterol: 57mg; Carbohydrates: 20g; Fiber: 6g; Protein: 26g; Sodium: 698mg

FOIL-BAKED SALMON WITH GREEK YOGURT CILANTRO SAUCE

GLUTEN-FREE

Serves 6 | Prep time: 10 minutes | Cook time: 20 minutes
Serving size: 3 ounces cooked salmon and ¼ cup sauce

This easy baked salmon will become a regular on the dinner rotation. In no time flat, prepare a Mediterranean-style dish blending flavors of lemon, garlic, and cilantro to delight your taste buds. Serve with grilled vegetables and whole-grain brown rice for a heart-healthy meal.

½ **salmon side (about 1½ pounds), skin on**

2 **tablespoons extra-virgin olive oil**

1 **teaspoon sea salt, divided**

½ **teaspoon freshly ground black pepper, divided**

1 **teaspoon ground coriander**

1 **teaspoon ground cumin**

Juice and zest of 1 lemon, divided

1½ **cups nonfat plain Greek yogurt**

¼ **cup chopped fresh cilantro**

1 **garlic clove, minced**

1. Preheat the oven to 375°F.
2. Place a large piece of aluminum foil (large enough to wrap the salmon, with room for liquid) on a rimmed baking sheet. Place the salmon, skin-side down, on the foil. Fold up and crimp the sides but leave the top open.
3. In a small bowl, whisk together the olive oil, ½ teaspoon of salt, ¼ teaspoon of pepper, the coriander, cumin, and lemon juice.
4. Pour over the salmon and seal the foil at the top.
5. Bake until the salmon is flaky and opaque, 15 to 20 minutes.
6. While the salmon cooks, in a small bowl, whisk together the Greek yogurt, cilantro, garlic, lemon zest, remaining ½ teaspoon of salt, and remaining ¼ teaspoon of pepper.
7. Serve the salmon with the sauce spooned over the top.

Variation tip: Replace the cilantro with chopped fresh dill, and replace the lemon juice with orange juice.

Per Serving: Calories: 247; Total fat: 9g; Saturated fat: 2g; Cholesterol: 75mg; Carbohydrates: 3g; Fiber: <1g; Protein: 35g; Sodium: 507mg

TROUT PUTTANESCA

GLUTEN-FREE

Serves 4 | Prep time: 10 minutes | Cook time: 15 minutes | Serving size: 1½ cups

Puttanesca, a word translated, roughly, to "lady of the night," is the name of a tasty sauce deliciously paired with one of the best fish sources of protein and omega-3s. Trout is known for its mild flavor and delicate texture—some even say it's comparable to eating a tender beefsteak.

2 tablespoons extra-virgin olive oil

1 pound trout, skinned and cut into 1-inch pieces

½ teaspoon sea salt

¼ teaspoon freshly ground black pepper

1 shallot, minced

3 garlic cloves, minced

1 (14-ounce) can chopped tomatoes, drained

1 tablespoon dried Italian seasoning

1 tablespoon capers, drained and rinsed

1 (5-ounce) can sliced black olives, drained

¼ teaspoon red pepper flakes

2 tablespoons chopped fresh basil

1. In a large skillet, heat the olive oil over medium-high heat until it shimmers.

2. Season the trout with the salt and black pepper. Put it in the skillet and cook, stirring occasionally, until flaky, about 6 minutes total.

3. Using a slotted spoon, remove the fish from the fat in the skillet and set aside on a platter.

4. Add the shallot and cook, stirring occasionally, until soft, about 3 minutes.

5. Add the garlic and cook, stirring constantly, for 30 seconds.

6. Add the tomatoes, Italian seasoning, capers, olives, and red pepper flakes. Cook, stirring, for 5 minutes. Return the trout to the pan and cook, stirring, for an additional 2 minutes.

7. Remove from the heat. Stir in the basil before serving.

Ingredient tip: Trout has lots of tiny pin bones. Before cutting the trout into pieces, use a magnifying glass and good light to find the bones, and use small, needle-nosed pliers to remove them.

Per Serving: Calories: 306; Total fat: 18g; Saturated fat: 3g; Cholesterol: 78mg; Carbohydrates: 8g; Fiber: 2g; Protein: 27g; Sodium: 703mg

PAN-SEARED TROUT WITH ORANGE-GARLIC SPINACH

GLUTEN-FREE

Serves 4 | Prep time: 10 minutes | Cook time: 15 minutes | Serving size: 1 trout fillet and ½ cup spinach

Whether bought at your local grocery store or caught on a fishing trip, this trout is divine eating. Seasoned subtly with garlic and fresh orange juice along with buttery, mildly sweet pine nuts, it's a mouthwatering marvel.

4 (4- to 6-ounce) trout fillets, skin on, pin bones removed

1 teaspoon sea salt, divided

½ teaspoon freshly ground black pepper, divided

3 tablespoons extra-virgin olive oil, divided

4 cups baby spinach

3 garlic cloves, minced

Juice of 1 orange

¼ cup pine nuts

1. Season the trout fillets with ½ teaspoon of salt and ¼ teaspoon of pepper.
2. In a large skillet, heat 2 tablespoons of olive oil over medium-high heat until it shimmers.
3. Place the trout in the pan, skin-side down, and cook without disturbing it until the skin is browned, about 4 minutes. Flip and cook on the other side until the trout is opaque, about 3 minutes more. Remove from the pan and set aside on a platter tented with foil to keep warm.
4. In the same pan, heat 1 tablespoon of olive oil.
5. Add the spinach, the remaining ½ teaspoon of salt, and the remaining ¼ teaspoon of pepper. Cook, stirring, until it wilts, about 2 minutes.
6. Add the garlic and cook, stirring constantly, for 30 seconds.
7. Add the orange juice. Cook, stirring, for 1 minute more.
8. Remove from the heat and add the pine nuts. Spoon the spinach and sauce over the trout, and serve.

Per Serving: Calories: 337; Total fat: 23g; Saturated fat: 4g; Cholesterol: 78mg; Carbohydrates: 5g; Fiber: 2g; Protein: 28g; Sodium: 680mg

CITRUS-MINT SALMON

GLUTEN-FREE

Serves 4 | Prep time: 10 minutes, plus 10 minutes to marinate | Cook time: 10 minutes
Serving size: 1 salmon fillet

Citrus and salmon are a perfectly matched dynamic duo. What you get is a tangy, slightly sweet flavor that pairs nicely with sugar snap peas or steamed broccoli and baby carrots. Better yet, salmon is the all-star of heart-healthy eating thanks to its abundance of omega-3 fatty acids, known to reduce blood pressure and keep clotting at bay.

½ cup freshly squeezed orange juice

1 tablespoon reduced-sodium Worcestershire sauce

½ teaspoon Dijon mustard

4 tablespoons extra-virgin olive oil, divided

2 tablespoons chopped fresh mint

4 (4-ounce) salmon fillets

1. In a shallow dish, whisk together the orange juice, Worcestershire sauce, mustard, 2 tablespoons of olive oil, and mint.
2. Place the salmon fillets flesh-side down in the marinade and allow them to rest for 10 minutes.
3. Remove the salmon from the marinade and pat dry.
4. In a large nonstick skillet, heat the remaining 2 tablespoons of olive oil over medium-high heat until it shimmers.
5. Place the salmon, flesh-side down, in the skillet. Cook, undisturbed, until the salmon browns, about 4 minutes.
6. Flip and continue to cook until cooked through, another 3 to 4 minutes. Serve.

Per Serving: Calories: 275; Total fat: 19g; Saturated fat: 3g; Cholesterol: 85mg; Carbohydrates: 4g; Fiber: <1g; Protein: 23g; Sodium: 105mg

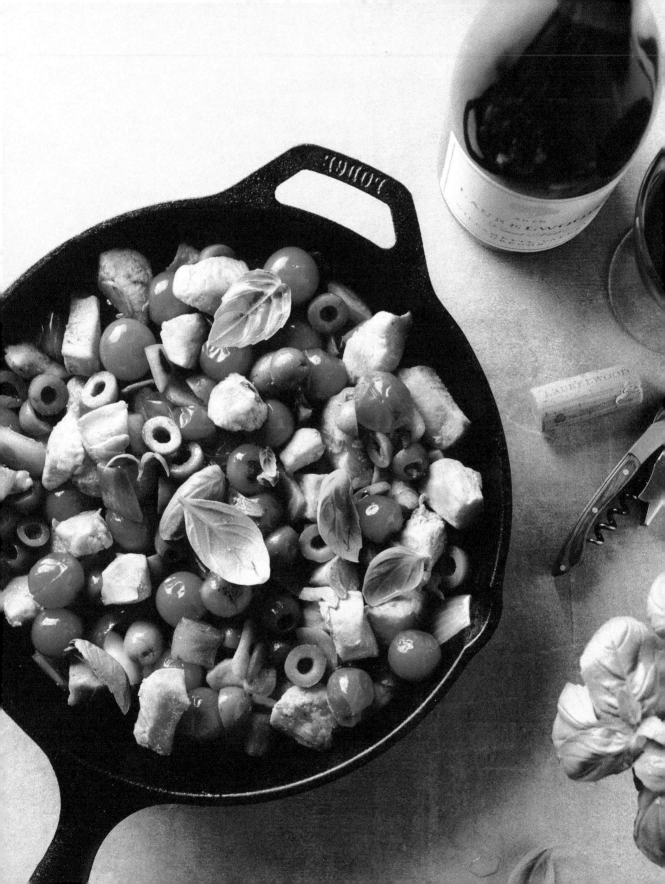

CHAPTER 8

POULTRY AND BEEF ENTRÉES

< *Skillet Chicken with Olives and Tomatoes,*
page 144

TURKEY PICCATA

Serves 4 | Prep time: 10 minutes | Cook time: 10 minutes | Serving size: 1 turkey cutlet

If you love veal or chicken sautéed in a sauce of lemon juice and capers, you'll be delighted with this recipe. Quick, easy, and scrumptious, turkey breasts take this dish to new culinary heights.

½ cup whole-wheat flour

½ teaspoon sea salt

¼ teaspoon freshly ground black pepper

4 (4-ounce) boneless, skinless turkey breast cutlets, pounded to ¼-inch thickness

2 tablespoons olive oil

½ cup dry white wine

½ shallot, minced

Juice of 2 lemons

2 tablespoons capers, drained and rinsed

1. In a shallow dish, whisk together the flour, salt, and pepper.
2. Dip the turkey cutlets in the flour mixture and shake off any excess.
3. In a large skillet, heat the olive oil over medium-high heat until it shimmers.
4. Place the turkey in the skillet and cook until browned, 1 to 2 minutes per side. Set the turkey aside on a platter tented with foil to keep warm.
5. In the same pan, add the wine, shallot, lemon juice, and capers, using the side of a spoon to scrape any browned bits from the bottom of the pan. Bring to a simmer. Cook until the liquid is reduced by half, about 3 minutes.
6. Return the turkey to the pan and turn it to coat with the sauce.
7. Serve with the sauce spooned over the turkey.

Substitution tip: Make this gluten-free by using gluten-free all-purpose flour.

Per Serving: Calories: 259; Total fat: 8g; Saturated fat: 1g; Cholesterol: 70mg; Carbohydrates: 14g; Fiber: 1g; Protein: 30g; Sodium: 418mg

SPAGHETTI WITH TURKEY BOLOGNESE

Serves 4 | Prep time: 10 minutes | Cook time: 15 minutes | Serving size: 1 cup pasta and ½ cup sauce

Originating from Bologna, Italy, Bolognese is an Italian favorite and a reminder that good food doesn't have to be complicated or use fancy ingredients. Choose packages labeled "ground turkey breasts," an excellent source of niacin and selenium. Using ground turkey makes for a lighter weeknight pasta sauce full of bold flavor. Invite friends over and relish in the rave reviews.

2 tablespoons extra-virgin olive oil

1 pound ground turkey

1 onion, chopped

2 carrots, peeled and chopped

3 garlic cloves, minced

1 (28-ounce) can crushed tomatoes

1 tablespoon dried Italian seasoning

½ teaspoon sea salt

Pinch red pepper flakes

8 ounces whole-wheat spaghetti, cooked according to package instructions and drained

1. In a large skillet, heat the olive oil over medium-high heat until it shimmers.

2. Add the turkey and cook, crumbling with a wooden spoon, until browned, about 5 minutes.

3. Add the onion and carrots and cook, stirring occasionally, until soft, about 5 minutes more.

4. Add the garlic and cook, stirring constantly, for 30 seconds.

5. Add the tomatoes with their juices, Italian seasoning, salt, and red pepper flakes. Bring to a simmer. Simmer, stirring occasionally, for 5 minutes more.

6. Spoon the sauce over the spaghetti and serve.

Nutritional boost: Pump up the heart-healthy nutrition by adding 1 cup of chopped kale in step 3.

Per Serving: Calories: 435; Total fat: 9g; Saturated fat: 1g; Cholesterol: 70mg; Carbohydrates: 48g; Fiber: 10g; Protein: 45g; Sodium: 641mg

MEDITERRANEAN-STYLE GROUND TURKEY AND VEGGIE SKILLET

ALLERGEN-FREE, GLUTEN-FREE

Serves 4 | Prep time: 10 minutes | Cook time: 10 minutes | Serving size: ¾ cup

Lean ground turkey with delicious flavors of delicately sweet and savory veggies is a hearty "welcome home" after a long day at work. Complete the meal with a side of cooked lentils added to whole-grain barley for a fiber and potassium boost.

2 tablespoons extra-virgin olive oil

1 pound ground turkey

1 onion, chopped

1 fennel bulb, sliced

1 (14-ounce) can artichoke bottoms, drained and chopped

1 pint cherry tomatoes

1 tablespoon dried Italian seasoning

½ teaspoon sea salt

¼ teaspoon freshly ground black pepper

4 garlic cloves, minced

1. In a large skillet, heat the olive oil over medium-high heat until it shimmers.
2. Add the turkey and cook, crumbling with a wooden spoon, until browned, about 5 minutes.
3. Add the onion, fennel, artichoke bottoms, tomatoes, Italian seasoning, salt, and pepper. Cook, stirring occasionally, until the vegetables soften, about 5 minutes.
4. Add the garlic and cook, stirring, for 30 seconds.
5. Serve.

Ingredient tip: To add bright flavors, garnish with a squeeze of fresh lemon juice and ¼ cup of chopped fresh Italian parsley.

Per Serving: Calories: 263; Total fat: 9g; Saturated fat: 1g; Cholesterol: 70mg; Carbohydrates: 18g; Fiber: 6g; Protein: 32g; Sodium: 639mg

TURKEY AND FARRO STUFFED BELL PEPPERS

Serves 4 | Prep time: 15 minutes | Cook time: 1 hour | Serving size: 1 pepper and ½ cup filling

If you love stuffed peppers, you must make this appetizing recipe. Kudos to farro! This ancient grain provides lots of heart-health benefits due to being a rich source of fiber, iron, protein, and magnesium.

2 tablespoons extra-virgin olive oil

1 pound ground turkey

1 onion, chopped

4 cups chopped kale

4 garlic cloves, minced

1 (15-ounce) can crushed tomatoes, drained

1 tablespoon dried Italian seasoning

2 cups cooked farro

½ teaspoon sea salt

⅛ teaspoon freshly ground black pepper

4 red bell peppers, tops cut off, seeded

½ cup crumbled feta cheese

1. Preheat the oven to 350°F. Line a rimmed baking sheet with parchment paper and set aside.
2. In a large skillet, heat the olive oil over medium-high heat until it shimmers.
3. Add the turkey and cook, crumbling with a wooden spoon, until browned, about 5 minutes.
4. Add the onion and kale and cook, stirring occasionally, until the vegetables soften, about 5 minutes.
5. Add the garlic and cook, stirring, for 30 seconds.
6. Add the tomatoes and Italian seasoning and cook, stirring occasionally, for 5 minutes. Stir in the cooked farro, salt, and black pepper. Cook for 2 minutes more.
7. Spoon the mixture into the bell peppers and place them on the prepared baking sheet. Sprinkle with the feta cheese.
8. Bake until the peppers are soft, about 40 minutes. Serve.

Substitution tip: **Make this gluten-free by replacing the farro with 2 cups of cooked brown rice.**

Per Serving: Calories: 434; Total fat: 14g; Saturated fat: 4g; Cholesterol: 87mg; Carbohydrates: 49g; Fiber: 10g; Protein: 42g; Sodium: 720mg

GROUND TURKEY AND RICE SKILLET

ALLERGEN-FREE, GLUTEN-FREE

Serves 4 | Prep time: 15 minutes | Cook time: 20 minutes | Serving size: 1½ cups

There are certain recipes we cook over and over because they use basic ingredients, are easy to make, and, bottom line, taste great. This Mediterranean-inspired rice dish adds nutrient- and fiber-rich veggies and lean ground turkey to the checklist for good cardiovascular health.

2 tablespoons extra-virgin olive oil

1 pound ground turkey

1 red onion, chopped

1 medium zucchini, chopped

1 pint grape tomatoes, halved

½ cup sliced black olives

3 garlic cloves, minced

Juice of 1 lemon

1 teaspoon ground oregano

½ teaspoon sea salt

¼ teaspoon freshly ground black pepper

2 cups cooked brown rice

1. In a large skillet, heat the olive oil over medium-high heat until it shimmers.
2. Add the turkey and cook, crumbling with a wooden spoon, until browned, about 5 minutes.
3. Add the onion and zucchini and cook, stirring occasionally, until the vegetables soften, about 5 minutes. Add the tomatoes and olives and cook, stirring, for 2 minutes more.
4. Add the garlic and cook, stirring, for 30 seconds.
5. Add the lemon juice, oregano, salt, pepper, and rice and cook, stirring occasionally, until the rice is warmed through, about 4 minutes. Serve.

Variation tip: Garnish this with ½ cup of crumbled feta cheese and ¼ cup of chopped fresh Italian parsley.

Per Serving: Calories: 355; Total fat: 12g; Saturated fat: 1g; Cholesterol: 70mg; Carbohydrates: 33g; Fiber: 4g; Protein: 32g; Sodium: 485mg

TURKEY MEATLOAF MUFFINS

Serves 4 | Prep time: 15 minutes | Cook time: 30 minutes | Serving size: 3 muffins

There's one word for this meal: *wow*. This isn't your mama's meatloaf. Spicy, meaty, and satisfying, when served with a mix of sautéed or steamed nutrient-rich broccoli, cauliflower, and peppers on the side, this meal pops with tantalizing flavors.

½ cup skim milk

½ cup whole-wheat bread crumbs

2 tablespoons olive oil

1 onion, chopped

3 garlic cloves, minced

8 ounces ground turkey

8 ounces ground Italian turkey sausage

1 egg, beaten

1 tablespoon dried Italian seasoning

½ teaspoon sea salt

Nonstick cooking spray

1. Preheat the oven to 350°F.
2. In a large bowl, combine the milk and bread crumbs. Allow to sit for 10 minutes.
3. Meanwhile, in a large skillet, heat the olive oil over medium-high heat until it shimmers.
4. Add the onion and cook, stirring occasionally, until soft, about 3 minutes.
5. Add the garlic and cook, stirring, for 30 seconds. Cool slightly.
6. In the bowl with the milk and bread crumbs, add the turkey, Italian turkey sausage, egg, Italian seasoning, salt, and cooked onions and garlic. Mix well.
7. Spray a 12-cup muffin tin with cooking spray, and spoon the meatloaf mixture into each cup.
8. Bake until the internal temperature reads 165°F, about 25 minutes. Serve.

Substitution tip: Make this gluten-free by replacing the bread crumbs with ½ cup of almond flour.

Per Serving: Calories: 287; Total fat: 13g; Saturated fat: 3g; Cholesterol: 122mg; Carbohydrates: 15g; Fiber: 1g; Protein: 24g; Sodium: 661mg

TUSCAN-STYLE CHICKEN STEW

ALLERGEN-FREE, GLUTEN-FREE

Serves 4 | Prep time: 15 minutes | Cook time: 25 minutes | Serving size: 1 cup

If you've been searching for Tuscan-style cuisine evoking the feel of the Mediterranean, this recipe, made with simple ingredients, is for you. Feel free to add some canned cannellini beans and chopped carrots for an even heartier weeknight meal.

3 tablespoons extra-virgin olive oil, divided

1 pound boneless, skinless chicken breast, cut into 1-inch cubes

1 onion, chopped

5 garlic cloves, sliced

½ cup dry white wine

1 (28-ounce) can crushed tomatoes, drained

1 tablespoon dried Italian seasoning

1 cup Spanish olives, pitted and halved

½ teaspoon sea salt

¼ teaspoon red pepper flakes

1. In a large pot, heat 2 tablespoons of olive oil over medium-high heat until it shimmers.
2. Add the chicken and cook, stirring occasionally, until browned, about 8 minutes. Remove the chicken and set it aside.
3. Add the remaining 1 tablespoon of olive oil to the pot. Add the onion and garlic and cook, stirring occasionally, until soft, 3 to 4 minutes.
4. Add the white wine, using the side of a spoon to scrape any browned bits from the bottom of the pan.
5. Add the tomatoes, Italian seasoning, olives, salt, and red pepper flakes. Return the chicken to the pot.
6. Bring to a simmer, reduce the heat, and continue to simmer, stirring occasionally, for 10 minutes. Serve.

Ingredient tip: Add fresh flavors by garnishing this with 2 tablespoons each of chopped fresh basil and Italian parsley.

Per Serving: Calories: 321; Total fat: 17g; Saturated fat: 3g; Cholesterol: 65mg; Carbohydrates: 12g; Fiber: 3g; Protein: 31g; Sodium: 1,111mg

EASY ROTINI AND CHICKEN BAKE

Serves 4 | Prep time: 15 minutes | Cook time: 55 minutes | Serving size: 1 cup pasta and ½ cup sauce

Think of this as your "ready, set, eat" meal. Dinner comes together in no time, and with lean ground chicken, fresh veggies, spices, and pasta, this dish will satisfy even the pickiest of eaters.

Nonstick cooking spray

2 tablespoons extra-virgin olive oil

1 pound ground chicken breast

1 onion, chopped

2 cups chopped kale

2 garlic cloves, minced

1 (28-ounce) can crushed tomatoes, drained

1 tablespoon dried Italian seasoning

½ teaspoon sea salt

8 ounces whole-wheat rotini pasta, cooked according to package instructions and drained

½ cup shredded Parmesan cheese

1. Preheat the oven to 350°F. Spray a 9-by-13-inch baking dish with nonstick cooking spray and set aside.

2. In a large skillet, heat the olive oil over medium-high heat until it shimmers.

3. Add the chicken and cook, crumbling with a wooden spoon, until browned, about 5 minutes.

4. Add the onion and kale and cook, stirring occasionally, until the onion is soft, about 4 minutes.

5. Add the garlic and cook, stirring constantly, for 30 seconds.

6. Add the tomatoes, Italian seasoning, and salt. Bring to a simmer and cook, stirring, for 5 minutes. Stir in the rotini.

7. Pour the mixture into the prepared baking dish. Sprinkle evenly with the Parmesan cheese.

8. Bake for 40 minutes. Let cool slightly before serving.

Per serving: Calories: 534; Total fat: 22g; Saturated fat: 5g; Cholesterol: 118mg; Carbohydrates: 56g; Fiber: 10g; Protein: 41g; Sodium: 904mg

CHERMOULA CHICKEN WITH COUSCOUS

Serves 4 | Prep time: 15 minutes, plus 8 hours to marinate | Cook time: 25 minutes
Serving size: 1 chicken breast and ½ cup couscous

Marinated chicken breasts are always good, but when made "chermoula-style," they become fabulous Moroccan-inspired creations featuring garlic, lemon, and warm spices. The flavors blend beautifully, pairing exceptionally well with a side of herbed couscous mixed with pine nuts.

Juice of 3 lemons

¼ cup extra-virgin olive oil

1 teaspoon ground cumin

1 tablespoon paprika

4 garlic cloves, minced

½ teaspoon sea salt

½ cup chopped fresh cilantro, divided

4 (4- to 6-ounce) boneless, skinless chicken breasts

½ cup uncooked whole-wheat couscous

¼ cup pine nuts

1. In a blender, combine the lemon juice, olive oil, cumin, paprika, garlic, salt, and ¼ cup of cilantro. Blend until smooth.
2. Pour into a zip-top bag, add the chicken breasts, seal the bag, and let the chicken marinate in the refrigerator for 8 hours.
3. Preheat the oven to 400°F. Line a baking dish with parchment paper.
4. Transfer the marinated chicken to the prepared baking dish.
5. Bake until the chicken reaches an internal temperature of 165°F, about 25 minutes.
6. While the chicken cooks, prepare the couscous according to the package instructions.
7. Stir the remaining ¼ cup of cilantro and the pine nuts into the couscous just before serving.
8. Serve the chicken with the herbed couscous on the side.

Substitution tip: Replace the couscous with ½ cup (per serving) of cooked brown rice or quinoa to make this gluten-free.

Per Serving: Calories: 398; Total fat: 22g; Saturated fat: 3g; Cholesterol: 65mg; Carbohydrates: 25g; Fiber: 3g; Protein: 28g; Sodium: 481mg

ARROZ CON POLLO

ALLERGEN-FREE, GLUTEN-FREE

Serves 4 | **Prep time: 15 minutes** | **Cook time: 15 minutes** | **Serving size: 1½ cups**

Let's just call this the perfect weeknight dinner. This traditional one-pot meal popular in Spain comes together easily and quickly. The flavor is so good, it'll be at the top of your recipe list.

2 tablespoons extra-virgin olive oil

1 pound boneless, skinless chicken breast, cut into 1-inch pieces

1 onion, chopped

1 teaspoon paprika

3 garlic cloves, minced

½ cup dry white wine

1 (12-ounce) jar roasted red peppers, drained and chopped

2 cups fresh or frozen peas

2 cups cooked brown rice

1. In a large skillet, heat the olive oil over medium-high heat until it shimmers.

2. Add the chicken and cook until browned, about 7 minutes.

3. Add the onion and paprika and cook until soft, another 3 to 4 minutes.

4. Add the garlic and cook, stirring constantly, for 30 seconds.

5. Add the wine and use the side of a spoon to scrape any browned bits from the bottom of the pan. Add the roasted red peppers, peas, and rice. Cook, stirring, until everything is heated through, about 4 minutes more. Serve.

Per Serving: Calories: 393; Total fat: 11g; Saturated fat: 2g; Cholesterol: 65mg; Carbohydrates: 41g; Fiber: 7g; Protein: 30g; Sodium: 328mg

CHICKEN WITH WHITE WINE, MUSHROOMS, AND ORZO

Serves 4 | Prep time: 15 minutes | Cook time: 25 minutes | Serving size: 1½ cups

Here's what great heart-healthy eating is all about. Lean chicken breast and veggies tossed with whole-grain orzo is a comfort-food dish that goes great with a crunchy side salad.

3 tablespoons extra-virgin olive oil, divided

4 slices turkey bacon, chopped

1 pound boneless, skinless chicken breast, cut into 1-inch cubes

1 shallot, minced

8 ounces cremini mushrooms, sliced

1 teaspoon dried thyme

½ teaspoon sea salt

¼ teaspoon freshly ground black pepper

3 garlic cloves, minced

2 tablespoons whole-wheat flour

2 cups dry white wine

1 cup whole-wheat orzo, cooked according to package instructions and drained

1. In a large skillet, heat 2 tablespoons of olive oil over medium-high heat until it shimmers.
2. Add the turkey bacon and cook until browned, about 5 minutes. Using a slotted spoon, remove the bacon from the fat and set aside.
3. Add the chicken to the rendered fat in the skillet and cook, stirring occasionally, until browned, about 7 minutes. Remove from the pan and set aside.
4. In the same skillet, add the remaining 1 tablespoon of olive oil and heat until it shimmers.
5. Add the shallot, mushrooms, thyme, salt, and pepper. Cook, stirring occasionally, until the mushrooms are deeply browned, 6 to 7 minutes.
6. Add the garlic and cook, stirring, for 30 seconds.
7. Add the flour and cook, stirring, for 30 seconds more.
8. Add the wine, using the side of a spoon to scrape any browned bits from the bottom of the pan. Return the chicken and bacon to the pan. Cook, stirring occasionally, until the sauce is thick and everything is heated through, about 4 minutes more.
9. Toss with the hot orzo and serve.

Per Serving: Calories: 548; Total fat: 17g; Saturated fat: 3g; Cholesterol: 75mg; Carbohydrates: 50g; Fiber: 7g; Protein: 34g; Sodium: 615mg

ROASTED CHICKEN THIGHS WITH POTATOES AND FENNEL

ALLERGEN-FREE, GLUTEN-FREE

Serves 4 | Prep time: 15 minutes | Cook time: 1 hour
Serving size: 1 chicken thigh and 1 cup vegetables

Chicken thighs have never tasted so good thanks to fennel, a perennial aromatic herb. Popularly used in Mediterranean cooking, fennel has unique health benefits from the flavonoids quercetin and rutin, both potent antioxidants that may reduce inflammation to help prevent heart disease.

4 bone-in, skin-on chicken thighs

¾ teaspoon sea salt, divided

¼ teaspoon freshly ground black pepper

2 teaspoons dried tarragon, divided

2 fennel bulbs, thinly sliced

20 baby potatoes, halved

2 tablespoons extra-virgin olive oil

1. Preheat the oven to 400°F.
2. Season the chicken with ¼ teaspoon of salt, the pepper, and 1 teaspoon of tarragon.
3. In a large bowl, combine the fennel, baby potatoes, olive oil, remaining ½ teaspoon of salt, and remaining 1 teaspoon of tarragon. Toss to mix.
4. Spread the fennel and potatoes in a 9-by-13-inch baking dish. Arrange the chicken on top.
5. Bake until the chicken reaches an internal temperature of 165°F, about 1 hour. Serve.

Per Serving: Calories: 428; Total fat: 26g; Saturated fat: 6g; Cholesterol: 111mg; Carbohydrates: 27g; Fiber: 6g; Protein: 23g; Sodium: 515mg

SKILLET CHICKEN WITH OLIVES AND TOMATOES

ALLERGEN-FREE, GLUTEN-FREE

Serves 4 | Prep time: 10 minutes | Cook time: 15 minutes | Serving size: 1½ cups

You'll find plenty of heart-healthy support in this dish. Lean chicken breast, olives brimming with healthy monounsaturated fat, and antioxidant-rich herbs and spices make this a hands-down winner toward helping dodge heart disease.

2 tablespoons extra-virgin olive oil

1 pound boneless, skinless chicken breast, cut into 1-inch pieces

1 red onion, chopped

2 cups Spanish olives, pitted and halved

1 pint cherry tomatoes

3 garlic cloves, sliced

¼ cup chopped fresh basil

1. In a large skillet, heat the olive oil over medium-high heat until it shimmers.
2. Add the chicken and cook, stirring, until browned, about 7 minutes.
3. Add the onion and cook until soft, about 3 minutes. Add the olives, tomatoes, and garlic. Cook, stirring occasionally, until the tomatoes are soft, about 5 minutes more.
4. Serve garnished with the basil.

Nutritional boost: Add a helping of heart-healthy greens by stirring in 3 cups of baby spinach when you add the olives and tomatoes.

Per Serving: Calories: 294; Total fat: 17g; Saturated fat: 3g; Cholesterol: 65mg; Carbohydrates: 7g; Fiber: 2g; Protein: 24g; Sodium: 938mg

BEEF PINWHEELS WITH SPINACH AND GOAT CHEESE

GLUTEN-FREE

**Serves 6 | Prep time: 10 minutes, plus 10 minutes to rest | Cook time: 30 minutes
Serving size: 1 pinwheel**

Research has shown you can enjoy portioned-controlled lean cuts of beef when eating for a healthy heart. This super-flavorful and tasty meal, along with a generous helping of fiber- and potassium-rich veggies, can be what to have for dinner tonight.

1½ pounds beef loin roast, butterflied and pounded to ½-inch thickness (see Ingredient tip)

½ teaspoon sea salt

¼ teaspoon freshly ground black pepper

1 (12-ounce) jar roasted red peppers, drained

2 (10-ounce) boxes frozen spinach, thawed

½ cup crumbled feta cheese

¼ cup pine nuts

1. Preheat the oven to 400°F.
2. Season the roast with the salt and black pepper.
3. Lay the roasted red peppers in a single layer on top of the meat. Cover with the spinach in an even layer. Sprinkle with the feta cheese and pine nuts.
4. Roll up the beef tightly and tie with butcher's twine. Place on a rimmed baking sheet.
5. Bake until the beef reaches an internal temperature of 145°F, about 30 minutes.
6. Let the roast rest for 10 minutes before cutting it into 6 pinwheels. Serve.

Ingredient tip: To butterfly the meat, use a sharp knife to cut straight down the middle of the beef from the top, leaving about ½ inch of meat uncut. Then, starting from the center opening and holding your knife parallel to the work surface, cut a slit outward to one side until your knife is ½ inch from the edge. Do the same on the other side of the center opening. Unfold the beef like a book and use a mallet to pound it to an even thickness.

Per Serving: Calories: 294; Total fat: 13g; Saturated fat: 4g; Cholesterol: 106mg; Carbohydrates: 9g; Fiber: 3g; Protein: 39g; Sodium: 490mg

CAPRESE BEEF

GLUTEN-FREE

Serves 4 | Prep time: 10 minutes | Cook time: 30 minutes | Serving size: 1 cup

Oh yes, this recipe is excellent eating. This dish marries some of the most notable ingredients in Italian cuisine: mozzarella, basil, olive oil, and tomatoes. Add lean, tender tri-tip beef, and you'll savor and revel in this delightful meal.

2 tablespoons extra-virgin olive oil

1 pound tri-tip steak, cut into 1-inch cubes

½ teaspoon sea salt

¼ teaspoon freshly ground black pepper

1 pint cherry tomatoes, halved

1 garlic clove, minced

½ cup shredded mozzarella cheese

¼ cup chopped fresh basil

1. In a large skillet, heat the olive oil over medium-high heat until it shimmers.
2. Add the steak, salt, and pepper and cook, stirring occasionally, until browned on all sides, about 20 minutes total.
3. Add the tomatoes and cook, stirring occasionally, for 5 minutes.
4. Add the garlic and cook, stirring, for 30 seconds.
5. Spread in an even layer on the bottom of the skillet and turn off the heat. Sprinkle evenly with the cheese. Cover and allow the cheese to melt, 3 to 4 minutes.
6. Sprinkle with the basil and serve.

Ingredient tip: If you can find it, fresh mozzarella (it comes packaged in water) is perfect for this recipe. Otherwise, shredded mozzarella is fine.

Per Serving: Calories: 402; Total fat: 25g; Saturated fat: 8g; Cholesterol: 84mg; Carbohydrates: 5g; Fiber: 1g; Protein: 39g

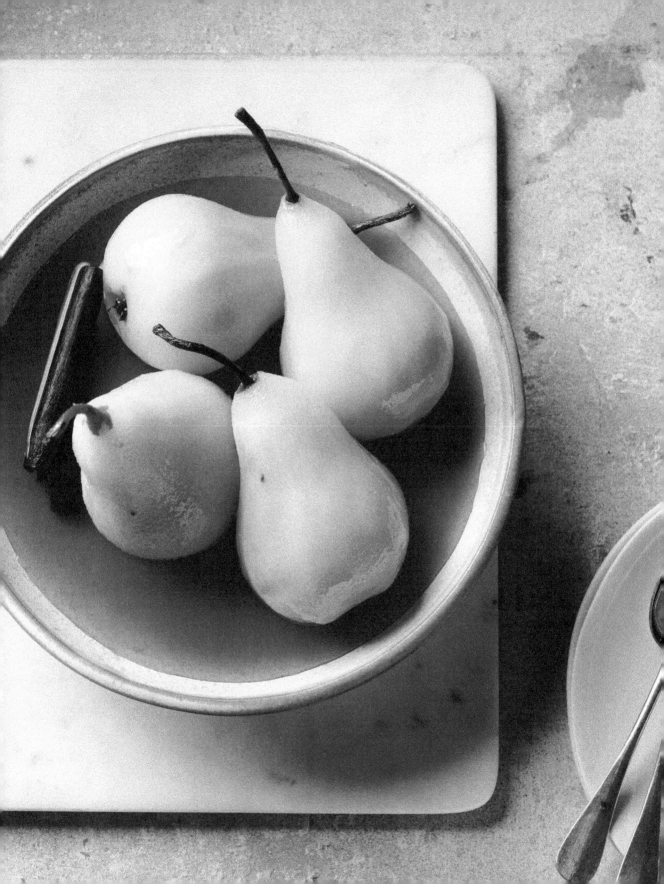

SWEET TREATS

*< Maple-Poached Pears,
page 155*

HONEY YOGURT PARFAITS WITH WALNUTS

GLUTEN-FREE, VEGETARIAN

Serves 4 | Prep time: 10 minutes | Serving size: 1 parfait

Whether eaten as an easy, on-the-go breakfast or as a nutritious snack, protein-packed Greek yogurt is always a healthy choice. Honey adds the perfect touch of sweetness, while the antioxidant-rich berries and omega-3-rich walnuts are a deliciously divine duo.

2 cups nonfat plain Greek yogurt

¼ cup honey

Juice of 1 orange

½ teaspoon pure vanilla extract

½ teaspoon ground cinnamon

1 pint raspberries

½ cup chopped walnuts

1. In a medium bowl, whisk together the yogurt, honey, orange juice, vanilla, and cinnamon.
2. Divide the raspberries among four tall glasses or parfait glasses. Layer each with ¼ cup of the yogurt mixture and 1 tablespoon of walnuts. Repeat these layers one more time. Serve.

Nutritional boost: Replace the raspberries with 2 cups of pomegranate seeds, which are high in antioxidants.

Per Serving: Calories: 266; Total fat: 10g; Saturated fat: 1g; Cholesterol: 0mg; Carbohydrates: 34g; Fiber: 6g; Protein: 14g; Sodium: 46mg

GREEK YOGURT CHOCOLATE MOUSSE

GLUTEN-FREE, VEGETARIAN

Serves 4 | Prep time: 10 minutes, plus 1 hour to chill | Serving size: ½ cup

Satisfy your chocolate cravings with this light and airy mousse. While a fancy French dessert such as mousse may sound intimidating, this one's a piece of cake to make. Whether you use maple syrup or amaretto liqueur to flavor it (see Variation tip), each lends its own unique, delicious note.

¼ **cup skim milk**

Zest of ½ orange

2 tablespoons pure maple syrup

1 teaspoon vanilla extract

1 cup semisweet chocolate chips, chopped

1 cup nonfat plain Greek yogurt

1. In a small saucepan, heat the milk, orange zest, and maple syrup over medium-high heat, stirring constantly, until it simmers. Remove from the heat and stir in the vanilla.

2. Put the chocolate chips in a medium bowl and pour the hot milk mixture over the top. Stir until the chocolate is melted and smooth. Let cool.

3. In another large bowl, whisk the Greek yogurt to ensure it's smooth. Fold in the cooled chocolate mixture.

4. Chill in the refrigerator for 1 hour before serving.

Variation tip: Replace the maple syrup with 2 tablespoons of amaretto liqueur. This will add a delicious almond note to the mousse.

Per Serving: Calories: 348; Total fat: 16g; Saturated fat: 10g; Cholesterol: <1mg; Carbohydrates: 46g; Fiber: <1g; Protein: 6g; Sodium: 30mg

YOGURT AND BERRY FREEZER POPS

GLUTEN-FREE, VEGETARIAN

Serves 4 | Prep time: 5 minutes, plus 6 hours to freeze | Serving size: 1 freezer pop

Remember how much you loved ice pops as a kid? Here's the healthier and tastier grown-up version—no guilt here. Calcium- and protein-packed, anti-inflammatory berries are jammed in this frozen treat, which is ideal for breakfast or as a midafternoon pick-me-up.

1 pint fresh blueberries or blackberries

½ cup nonfat plain Greek yogurt

2 tablespoons honey

2 cups skim milk

1. In a blender or food processor, combine the blueberries, yogurt, honey, and milk. Blend until smooth.
2. Pour into four ice pop molds.
3. Freeze for at least 6 hours before serving.

Ingredient tip: If you don't have ice pop molds, you can pour the mixture into paper cups and cover with aluminum foil. Insert ice pop sticks through the foil, which will hold them in place, and freeze. To serve, peel the cups and foil away from the frozen pops.

Per Serving: Calories: 130; Total fat: <1g; Saturated fat: <1g; Cholesterol: 3mg; Carbohydrates: 26g; Fiber: 2g; Protein: 7g; Sodium: 68mg

WARM APPLE COMPOTE WITH MAPLE CREAM

ALLERGEN-FREE, GLUTEN-FREE, VEGETARIAN

Serves 4 | Prep time: 10 minutes | Cook time: 20 minutes | Serving size: ½ cup apples and ¼ cup yogurt

Can't you just imagine how wonderfully tasty this warm compote will be? Substituting nonfat Greek yogurt for high-fat ice cream is smart for obtaining a calcium- and protein-packed punch of nutritional goodness. Top it off with heart-healthy nuts for some crunch.

6 sweet-tart apples (such as Honeycrisp), peeled, cored, and chopped

½ teaspoon ground cinnamon

½ teaspoon ground ginger

½ cup water

Pinch salt

6 tablespoons pure maple syrup, divided

1 cup nonfat plain Greek yogurt

1. In a large pot, combine the apples, cinnamon, ginger, water, salt, and 2 tablespoons of maple syrup. Bring to a simmer. Cover and cook, stirring occasionally, until the apples soften, about 20 minutes.

2. In a bowl, whisk together the Greek yogurt and the remaining 4 tablespoons of maple syrup.

3. Serve the compote warm or cold, topped with the maple cream.

Nutritional boost: Add heart-healthy fats by sprinkling each serving with 2 tablespoons of chopped walnuts or almonds.

Per Serving: Calories: 220; Total fat: <1g; Saturated fat: 0g; Cholesterol: 0mg; Carbohydrates: 51g; Fiber: 5g; Protein: 6g; Sodium: 45mg

GREEK YOGURT WITH GINGER-CRANBERRY COMPOTE

ALLERGEN-FREE, GLUTEN-FREE, VEGETARIAN

Serves 4 | Prep time: 5 minutes | Cook time: 10 minutes
Serving size: ¼ cup cranberries and ½ cup yogurt

This colorful fruit compote can be enjoyed as part of a delicious ending to a great meal. Traditionally associated with the holidays, your heart will be thankful any time of year when you serve cranberries. These red jewels are known to promote good heart health by possibly improving blood pressure and cholesterol.

1 (8-ounce) bag fresh cranberries

1 teaspoon grated orange zest, plus ½ cup freshly squeezed orange juice

1½ cups water, divided

¼ cup honey, plus 2 tablespoons honey

1 teaspoon ground ginger

3 tablespoons cornstarch

1 cup nonfat plain Greek yogurt

1. In a large, nonreactive pot, combine the cranberries, orange zest, 1¼ cups of water, orange juice, ¼ cup of honey, and ginger. Cook, stirring occasionally, over medium-high heat until the cranberries pop, about 8 minutes.
2. In a small bowl, whisk together the remaining ¼ cup of water and the cornstarch. Pour it into the simmering berries as you stir. Simmer, stirring, until thick, about 3 minutes more. Let cool.
3. In a bowl, whisk together the Greek yogurt and the remaining 2 tablespoons of honey.
4. Serve the yogurt with the cranberry compote spooned over the top.

Per Serving: Calories: 195; Total fat: <1g; Saturated fat: 0g; Cholesterol: 0mg; Carbohydrates: 44g; Fiber: 3g; Protein: 6g; Sodium: 25mg

MAPLE-POACHED PEARS

ALLERGEN-FREE, GLUTEN-FREE, VEGAN

Serves 4 | **Prep time: 5 minutes** | **Cook time: 20 minutes** | **Serving size: 1 pear**

Simple, elegant, and perfectly delicious, a fiber-rich stewed pear is also one of the healthiest desserts you can serve after a meal. Maple syrup gives a natural touch of sweetness to satisfy your craving for a sugary confection.

2 cups water

½ cup pure maple syrup

2 cinnamon sticks

4 pears, peeled

1. In a large pot, bring the water, maple syrup, and cinnamon sticks to a boil.
2. Add the pears. Bring back to a boil, then reduce the heat to medium. Cover and simmer until the pears are soft, about 20 minutes.
3. Serve warm.

Variation tip: **Make red wine–poached pears by replacing 1 cup of the water with 1 cup of dry red wine and replacing the maple syrup with ¼ cup of honey.**

Per Serving: Calories: 183; Total fat: <1g; Saturated fat: 0g; Cholesterol: 0mg; Carbohydrates: 48g; Fiber: 4g; Protein: 1g; Sodium: 4mg

HONEY-GLAZED BAKED PEACHES WITH HAZELNUTS

GLUTEN-FREE, VEGETARIAN

Serves 4 | Prep time: 5 minutes | Cook time: 15 minutes | Serving size: 1 peach

A juicy, sweet peach is a favorite fruit of mine, and I guarantee after trying this recipe, it will become a favorite of yours, too. Stone fruits like peaches are good sources of vitamin C, fiber, and potassium. Hazelnuts are high in magnesium and vitamin E, which work hard for your heart.

4 peaches, pitted and halved

2 tablespoons extra-virgin olive oil

¼ cup honey

½ teaspoon ground cinnamon

½ cup chopped hazelnuts

1. Preheat the oven to 350°F.
2. In a 9-inch square baking pan, place the peaches cut-side up. Drizzle the olive oil and honey over the peaches and sprinkle with the cinnamon.
3. Bake until the peaches are soft, about 10 minutes. Flip the peaches over and bake for another 5 minutes.
4. Sprinkle with the hazelnuts to serve.

Substitution tip: If you're allergic to nuts, you can sprinkle the peaches with pepitas instead.

Per Serving: Calories: 258; Total fat: 16g; Saturated fat: 2g; Cholesterol: 0mg; Carbohydrates: 31g; Fiber: 4g; Protein: 3g; Sodium: 1mg

FROYO WITH BLUEBERRY SAUCE

GLUTEN-FREE, VEGETARIAN

Serves 4 | Prep time: 5 minutes | Cook time: 10 minutes
Serving size: ½ cup yogurt and ¼ cup blueberries

Here's a dessert offering antioxidants, calcium, and vitamin C; better yet, it has an outstanding flavorful essence. Zesty with lots of gusto, this blueberry sauce will become a family favorite.

½ cup freshly squeezed orange juice

½ cup water, divided

3 cups fresh blueberries

1 teaspoon ground cinnamon

2 tablespoons honey

1½ tablespoons cornstarch

2 cups vanilla frozen yogurt

1. In a nonreactive saucepan, combine the orange juice, ¼ cup of water, the blueberries, cinnamon, and honey. Bring to a simmer. Cook, stirring occasionally, until the berries burst and start to get mushy, about 8 minutes.

2. In a small bowl, whisk the remaining ¼ cup of water with the cornstarch. Stir into the simmering berries and cook, stirring, until the sauce thickens, about 2 minutes more.

3. Cool and serve over the frozen yogurt.

Variation tip: You can replace the blueberries with 3 cups of fresh blackberries.

Per Serving: Calories: 234; Total fat: 4g; Saturated fat: 3g; Cholesterol: 1mg; Carbohydrates: 48g; Fiber: 3g; Protein: 4g; Sodium: 70mg

HONEYED MASCARPONE YOGURT WITH DRIED APRICOTS

Serves 4 | Prep time: 5 minutes | Serving size: ½ cup

Like tiramisu? Then you'll love this decadent dessert using mascarpone, a luxurious Italian cream cheese. Within 5 minutes, you'll be captivated by the combination of tangy, luscious sweetness from each ingredient.

8 ounces
mascarpone cheese

1 cup nonfat plain
Greek yogurt

¼ cup honey

¼ cup freshly squeezed
orange juice

1 cup chopped dried apricots

2 tablespoons chopped
fresh mint

1. In a blender, combine the mascarpone, yogurt, honey, and orange juice. Blend until smooth.
2. Spoon into four bowls. Stir ¼ cup of the apricots into each and garnish with the mint before serving.

Per Serving: Calories: 423; Total fat: 24g; Saturated fat: 10g; Cholesterol: 80mg; Carbohydrates: 42g; Fiber: 3g; Protein: 7g; Sodium: 48mg

BLACKBERRY-THYME GRANITA

ALLERGEN-FREE, GLUTEN-FREE, VEGETARIAN

Serves 4 | Prep time: 5 minutes, plus 4 hours to freeze | Serving size: ¼ cup

Similar to sorbet, granita is an Italian frozen dessert made by hand. It's a delightfully crunchy, melt-in-your mouth fruit ice—sort of like eating snow. Elegant enough to serve at a dinner party, granita can be made with just about any fruit, especially berries or watermelon, and will captivate your fruit-loving taste buds.

4 cups fresh blackberries

¼ cup honey

Juice of 1 lime

1 tablespoon chopped fresh thyme

1. In a blender, combine the blackberries, honey, lime juice, and thyme. Blend until smooth.
2. Strain into a bowl through a fine-mesh strainer, pressing to extract as much juice as possible. Discard the solids.
3. Pour onto a rimmed 9-by-13-inch baking sheet.
4. Freeze for 4 hours, using a fork every 30 minutes to scrape the freezing liquid into a texture similar to shaved ice. Serve.

Variation tip: This recipe also works with 4 cups of raspberries.

Per Serving: Calories: 143; Total fat: 1g; Saturated fat: 0g; Cholesterol: 0mg; Carbohydrates: 36g; Fiber: 8g; Protein: 1g; Sodium: 1mg

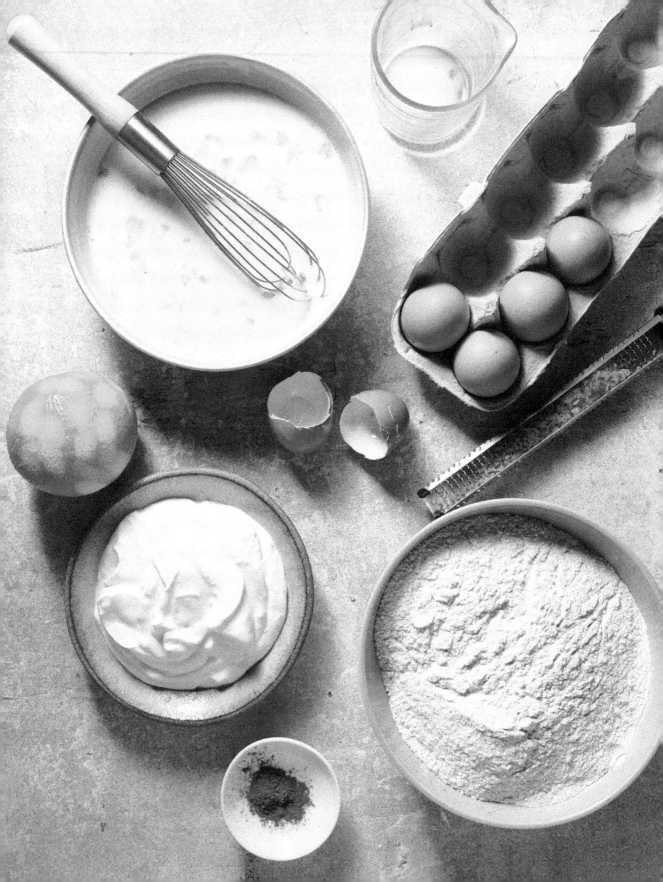

MEASUREMENT CONVERSIONS

VOLUME EQUIVALENTS (LIQUID)

US STANDARD	US STANDARD (OUNCES)	METRIC (APPROXIMATE)
2 tablespoons	1 fl. oz.	30 mL
¼ cup	2 fl. oz.	60 mL
½ cup	4 fl. oz.	120 mL
1 cup	8 fl. oz.	240 mL
1½ cups	12 fl. oz.	355 mL
2 cups or 1 pint	16 fl. oz.	475 mL
4 cups or 1 quart	32 fl. oz.	1 L
1 gallon	128 fl. oz.	4 L

VOLUME EQUIVALENTS (DRY)

US STANDARD	METRIC (APPROXIMATE)
⅛ teaspoon	0.5 mL
¼ teaspoon	1 mL
½ teaspoon	2 mL
¾ teaspoon	4 mL
1 teaspoon	5 mL
1 tablespoon	15 mL
¼ cup	59 mL
⅓ cup	79 mL
½ cup	118 mL
⅔ cup	156 mL
¾ cup	177 mL
1 cup	235 mL
2 cups or 1 pint	475 mL
3 cups	700 mL
4 cups or 1 quart	1 L

OVEN TEMPERATURES

FAHRENHEIT	CELSIUS (APPROXIMATE)
250°F	120° C
300°F	150° C
325°F	165° C
350°F	180° C
375°F	190° C
400°F	200° C
425°F	220° C
450°F	230° C

WEIGHT EQUIVALENTS

US STANDARD	METRIC (APPROXIMATE)
½ ounce	15 g
1 ounce	30 g
2 ounces	60 g
4 ounces	115 g
8 ounces	225 g
12 ounces	340 g
16 ounces or 1 pound	455 g

RESOURCES

Here are a few resources to help you and your loved ones learn more about heart disease and the Mediterranean diet:

Academy of Nutrition and Dietetics (EatRight.org): A national organization for registered dietitians in the United States that is the most credible source of nutrition information.

American Heart Association (Heart.org): A national organization in the United States that funds cardiovascular medical research; educates consumers on healthy living regarding diet, exercise, and stress management; and promotes cardiac care.

CardioSmart (CardioSmart.org): A patient education and empowerment initiative by the American College of Cardiology. Its mission is to help individuals prevent, treat, and manage cardiovascular disease.

Centers for Disease Control and Prevention (CDC.gov/heartdisease): A US federal agency that conducts and supports health promotion and prevention with the goal of improving public health.

Go Red for Women (GoRedForWomen.org): The American Heart Association's signature women's initiative that is a comprehensive platform designed to increase women's heart-health awareness and to serve as a catalyst for change to improve the lives of women globally.

Medline Plus: National Institutes of Health (MedlinePlus.gov): Produced by the National Library of Medicine, this website offers free, up-to-date, easily understandable information on diseases, such as heart disease. You can look up terms, view medical videos or illustrations, obtain the latest medical research on heart disease, and find out about clinical trials on a disease or condition.

Million Hearts (MillionHearts.hhs.gov): A national initiative to prevent one million heart attacks and strokes within five years. It focuses on implementing a small set of evidence-based priorities and targets that can improve cardiovascular health for all.

National Coalition for Women with Heart Disease (WomenHeart.org): The first national organization solely devoted to supporting women living with heart disease—the leading cause of death in women—and advocating and educating on their behalf.

National Heart, Lung, and Blood Institute (NHLBI.nih.gov): A national organization that develops education and awareness programs to effect positive change in public health. These initiatives focus on implementing national programs to help lower the risk for and consequences of heart, lung, blood, and sleep diseases and disorders.

Oldways (OldwaysPT.org): A nonprofit organization dedicated to helping people live healthy lives. It has a vast amount of information on Mediterranean diet plans and menus.

REFERENCES

American Heart Association. "Understand Your Risks to Prevent a Heart Attack." June 30, 2016. Heart.org/en/health-topics/heart-attack/understand-your-risks-to-prevent-a-heart-attack.

American Heart Association. "What Is Cardiovascular Disease?" May 31, 2017. Heart.org/en/health-topics/consumer-healthcare/what-is-cardiovascular-disease.

American Stroke Association. "About Stroke." February 15, 2017. Stroke.org/en/about-stroke.

Covenant HealthCare. "Types of Heart Disease." Accessed December 2, 2019. CovenantHealthCare.com/ch/typesofheartdisease.

Dietary Guidelines 2015–2020. "Appendix 4. USDA Food Patterns: Healthy Mediterranean-Style Eating Pattern." Accessed December 3, 2019. Health.gov/dietaryguidelines/2015/guidelines/appendix-4.

Estruch, Ramón, Emilio Ros, Jordi Salas-Salvadó, Maria-Isabel Covas, Dolores Corella, Fernando Arós, Enrique Gómez-Gracia, et al. "Primary Prevention of Cardiovascular Disease with a Mediterranean Diet." *New England Journal of Medicine* 386 (April 2013): 1279–90. doi:10.1056/NEJMoa1200303.

Estruch, Ramón, Emilio Ros, Jordi Salas-Salvadó, Maria-Isabel Covas, Dolores Corella, Fernando Arós, Enrique Gómez-Gracia, et al. "Primary Prevention of Cardiovascular Disease with a Mediterranean Diet Supplemented with Extra-Virgin Olive Oil or Nuts." *New England Journal of Medicine* 378 (June 2018): e34. doi:10.1056/NEJMoa1800389.

Gillinov, Marc, and Steven Nissen. "How Coronary Heart Disease Became Our Biggest Problem." *The Atlantic,* January 31, 2012. TheAtlantic.com/health/archive/2012/01/how-coronary-heart-disease-became-our-biggest-problem/251538.

Haseeb, Sohaib, Bryce Alexander, and Adrian Baranchuk. "Wine and Cardiovascular Health." *Circulation* 136, no. 15 (October 2017): 1434–48. doi:10.1161/CIRCULATIONAHA.117.030387.

Khera, Amit V., Connor A. Emdin, Isabel Drake, Pradeep Natarajan, Alexander G. Bick, Nancy R. Cook, Daniel I. Chasman, et al. "Genetic Risk, Adherence to a Healthy Lifestyle, and Coronary Disease." *New England Journal of Medicine* 375 (December 2016): 2349–58. doi:10.1056/NEJMoa1605086.

Kmietowicz, Zosia. "Fried Food Linked to Increased Risk of Death among Older US Women." *British Medical Journal* 364 (January 2019): 1362. doi:10.1136/bmj.l362.

Martínez-González, Miguel A., Alfredo Gea, and Miguel Ruiz-Canela. "The Mediterranean Diet and Cardiovascular Health." *Circulation Research* 124, no. 5 (February 2019): 779–98. AHAJournals.org/doi/full/10.1161/CIRCRESAHA.118.313348

McNeill, Shalene H. "Inclusion of Red Meat in Healthful Dietary Patterns." *Meat Science 98, no. 3* (November 2014): 452–60. doi:10.1016/j.meatsci.2014.06.028.

Qin, Chenxi, Jun Lv, Yu Guo, Zheng Bian, Jiahui Si, Ling Yang, Yiping Chen, et al. "Associations of Egg Consumption with Cardiovascular Disease in a Cohort Study of 0.5 Million Chinese Adults." *Heart* 104, no. 21 (November 2018): 1756–63. doi:10.1136/heartjnl-2017-312651.

Roussell, Michael A., Allison M. Hill, Trent L. Gaugler, Sheila G. West, John P. Vanden Heuvel, Peter Alaupovic, Peter J. Gillies, and Penny M. Kris-Etherton. "Beef in an Optimal Lean Diet Study: Effects on Lipids, Lipoproteins, and Apolipoproteins." *American Journal of Clinical Nutrition 95, no. 1* (January 2012): 9–16. doi:10.3945/ajcn.111.016261.

Sabate, Joan, Nasira M. Burkholder-Cooley, Gina Segovia-Siapco, Keiji Oda, Briana Wells, Michael J. Orlich, and Gary E. Fraser. "Unscrambling the Relations of Egg and Meat Consumption with Type 2 Diabetes Risk." *American Journal of Clinical Nutrition* 108, no. 5 (November 2018): 1121–28. doi:10.1093/ajcn/nqy213.

Saleem, T. S. Mohamed, and S. Darbar Basha. "Red Wine: A Drink to Your Heart." *Journal of Cardiovascular Disease Research* 1, no. 4 (October–December 2010): 171–76. doi:10.4103/0975-3583.74259.

Sanchez, Eduardo. "Life's Simple 7: Vital but Not Easy." *Journal of the American Heart Association* 7, no. 11 (May 2018): e009324. AHAJournals.org/doi/10.1161/JAHA.118.009324.

U.S. News and World Report. "U.S. News Reveals Best Diets Rankings for 2020." January 2, 2020. USNews.com/info/blogs/press-room/articles/2020-01-02/us-news-reveals-best-diets-rankings-for-2020

INDEX

ACKNOWLEDGMENTS

I am truly grateful for the unexpected yet welcomed opportunities I've been offered in my career as a registered dietitian. Writing books was only a dream at one time, but now, as a reality, it goes to show dreams really can come true. Without the support, advice, and encouragement of so many special individuals in my life, this dream would have fizzled long ago. At the top of my list, my husband, Casey, who is my rock and inspiration, always reassuring me to push ahead. I also extend my thanks and appreciation for the talents of my publishing team, Alyson Penn and Karen Frazier, along with the behind-the-scenes staff helping bring this book to life. My children, Peter, John, Liza, and Caroline, lovingly adored and for believing in their mom's pursuits. And to my extended family, friends, and colleagues, just knowing you cared meant the world to me.

ABOUT THE AUTHOR

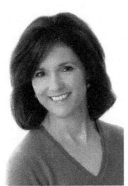

Cheryl Mussatto, MS, RD, LD, is a Kansas-based registered dietitian who holds a bachelor's degree in dietetics and institutional management from Kansas State University and a master's degree in dietetics and nutrition from the University of Kansas. Cheryl works at an endocrinology clinic, where she has counseled more than 1,500 patients, and is an adjunct professor at a community college and a freelance writer. She is the author of two books, *The Nourished Brain: The Latest Science on Food's Power for Protecting the Brain from Alzheimer's and Dementia* and *The Prediabetes Action Plan and Cookbook: A Simple Guide to Getting Healthy and Reversing Prediabetes*. Cheryl lives in northeast Kansas with her husband; they have four grown children. Visit her website at EatWellToBeWellRD.com.

CPSIA information can be obtained
at www.ICGtesting.com
Printed in the USA
LVHW010243191020
669099LV00007B/10